Mental Health Care for People with Learning Disabilities

For Churchill Livingstone:

Commissioning Editor: Susan Young
Project Editor: Catherine Jackson
Project Controller: Jane Dingwall
Designer: Judith Wright

Mental Health Care for People with Learning Disabilities

Helena Priest PhD MSc BA RN(MH) DipN DipNEd
Senior Lecturer, Keele University Department of Nursing and Midwifery,
Staffordshire, UK

Michael Gibbs MA RN(LD) PGCert CertEd
Lecturer, Keele University Department of Nursing and Midwifery,
Staffordshire, UK

Foreword by

Ruth Northway PhD MSc(Econ) RNLD CertEd(FE) FRCN
Professor of Learning Disability Nursing, University of Glamorgan, UK

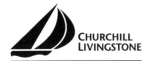
CHURCHILL
LIVINGSTONE

EDINBURGH LONDON NEW YORK OXFORD PHILADELPHIA ST LOUIS SYDNEY TORONTO 2004

CHURCHILL LIVINGSTONE
An imprint of Elsevier Limited

First published 2004

ISBN 0 443 07353 8

British Library Cataloguing in Publication Data
A catalogue record for this book is available from the British Library

Library of Congress Cataloging in Publication Data
A catalog record for this book is available from the Library of Congress

Notice
Medical knowledge is constantly changing. Standard safety
precautions must be followed, but as new research and clinical
experience broaden our knowledge, changes in treatment and drug
therapy may become necessary or appropriate. Readers are advised
to check the most current product information provided by the
manufacturer of each drug to be administered to verify the
recommended dose, the method and duration of administration, and
contraindications. It is the responsibility of the practitioner, relying on
experience and knowledge of the patient, to determine dosages and
the best treatment for each individual patient. Neither the Publisher
nor the authors assume any liability for any injury
and/or damage to persons or property arising from this publication.

The Publisher

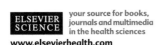
your source for books,
journals and multimedia
in the health sciences
www.elsevierhealth.com

The
Publisher's
policy is to use
**paper manufactured
from sustainable forests**

Printed in China

Contents

Contributor to Chapter 9

Peter Bates MA, CQSW
Senior Consultant, Mental Health and Learning Disabilities,
National Development Team, Manchester, UK

Foreword

For almost two decades there has been a growing awareness that the health needs of people with learning disabilities can often be unrecognised, unreported, and therefore untreated – this despite the fact that they experience the same health problems as other people (although sometimes with a different frequency) and that they can experience additional health problems as a result of their impairment (Welsh Health Planning Forum 1992).

In seeking to remedy this situation a number of barriers to health care have been identified. First, people with learning disabilities themselves may not recognise that any signs and symptoms they are experiencing are indicative of ill health. Even if there is such recognition, they may have difficulties in communicating this to others or in getting other people to listen, particularly where they have difficulties with verbal communication. This means that people with learning disabilities may be reliant upon others not only to recognise that they are experiencing ill health but also to recognise the importance of seeking appropriate help. However, family members and care staff may not be fully aware of the additional health needs which people with learning disabilities can experience.

A further barrier is diagnostic overshadowing, where any signs and symptoms are viewed as part of the learning disability rather than as being indicative of a health problem. Health professionals may also be unaware of specific health problems that are more prevalent amongst people with learning disabilities, and may lack the communication skills to derive important information from people with learning disabilities themselves or from their families and carers.

The fact that people with learning disabilities also experience mental ill health, and perhaps may experience such difficulties more frequently than other members of the population has, however, been slower to gain recognition than have their unmet physical health needs. Nonetheless a similar range of barriers to obtaining appropriate support is evident. Indeed some of these barriers may be compounded when considering mental ill health. For example, a characteristic of some forms of mental illness is that sufferers lack insight into their condition. Even if people with learning disabilities do recognise that they are experiencing difficulties with their mood, perceptions, or patterns of thinking this can be extremely difficult to communicate to others. It is more likely that any changes will be communicated via changes in behaviour, but others can interpret these as either part of the learning disability or as a form of challenging or 'difficult' behaviour.

This means that, in relation to meeting the mental health needs of people with learning disabilities, a number of things are essential. First there is a need for those involved in supporting people with learning disabilities to have an understanding of the causes and effects of various forms of mental health problems, to be aware of particular risk factors relating to people with learning disabilities, and to understand the need for good observational skills. Included in the group of people who need such awareness are family members, care staff, other people who may be involved in providing support (such as teachers), and health care staff.

Given that it can be difficult to detect the presence of mental ill health amongst people with learning disabilities then appropriate and accurate forms of assessment are required. It is also essential that such assessment leads to the development of packages of care which are monitored as to their effectiveness. A further key issue is the need to acknowledge that mental ill health is not an inevitability. Mental health promotion needs to be considered both in terms of prevention and in terms of promoting recovery.

This book is a welcome addition to the available literature since it seeks to address these issues in a format that is accessible to a range of key people who may be involved in supporting people with learning disabilities. The authors are to be commended for recognising and seeking to meet this need. It is to be hoped that it will be widely used and that its use will result in improved and enhanced services for people with learning disabilities who are suffering from, or who are at risk of, mental ill health.

Ruth Northway

REFERENCE

Welsh Health Planning Forum 1992 Protocol for investment in health gain – mental handicap (learning disabilities). Welsh Health Planning Forum, Cardiff

Preface

Mental health is a complex concept, and yet mental health problems are very common indeed. Most of us will, at some time in our life, experience stress and worry – at home, in education, or at work. We are also likely to feel sad or depressed from time to time. For each of us, however, the causes of these feelings will be different, the effects on our life will be different, and each of us will respond in our own unique ways. So what exactly is mental health, and what are mental health problems? What causes them? How do they affect individual lives? And, most importantly, in relation to this book, how do they affect the life of people with a learning disability, and those around them? In this book, we aim to answer these questions and, furthermore, to explore ways in which we can identify and respond to the mental health needs of clients with learning disabilities.

The notion that people with learning disabilities experience mental health problems is not new; in fact Menolascino discussed the idea as long ago as 1965. Today it is well documented that people with learning disabilities are at a higher risk of developing mental health problems than the general population. However, it is only in recent years that there has been a determined effort to address mental health assessment, diagnosis, services, education, and interventions for this client group.

Unfortunately, it seems that carers are sometimes limited in their understanding of mental health needs and in the skills and resources required to assess these needs and deliver appropriate care (Bates et al 2004, Gibbs & Priest 1999, Holt et al 2000, Quigley et al 2001). Although most professional and informal carers are generally well educated and very experienced, there has until recently been a shortage of specific educational provision to enable them to develop their knowledge, understanding and skill in the field of mental health as it relates to their client group.

This book is intended to go some way towards meeting these deficits. It is directed towards all those people, including parents and other family members, nurses, social workers, psychologists, occupational therapists, other professional staff, students, care staff, and voluntary workers, who are involved in the care of people with learning disabilities. The book does not profess to be a complete mental health manual. Rather, it aims to introduce the reader to the key issues and concerns that surround mental health in people with learning disabilities such that they might have a positive impact on the care that those people receive. The text is an introduction to the field and the authors would direct readers to material cited in the text for more in-depth analysis.

Each chapter focuses on a specific area. Chapter 1 provides the history, background, and context for the topic and introduces key concepts that are developed in subsequent chapters. Chapter 2 discusses a range of explanations for the occurrence of mental health problems, and how these might be relevant to people with learning disabilities. Chapter 3 considers the importance of assessment and discusses potential barriers to effective mental health assessment for people with learning disabilities. Chapter 4 introduces commonly occurring mental health problems, and their relevance to people with learning disabilities, while Chapter 5 outlines more specific syndromes and conditions that give rise to or mimic mental health problems. Chapter 6 provides an introduction to assessment tools, while Chapter 7 discusses interventions for mental health problems and their application in learning disability contexts. Chapter 8 focuses on mental health promotion, while Chapter 9 considers service provision for this client group. The book concludes, in Chapter 10, with a focus on the needs of the family in relation to learning disabilities and mental health problems. Chapters are supported by case studies and exercises that will help the reader to explore key concepts within the book. The case studies are fictitious, although based upon the authors' personal and professional experience, but in Chapter 10 we draw upon discussions carried out with actual clients and their families, whose names have been changed to protect their anonymity. Although the chapters can be read independently they also mesh to provide a foundation of knowledge in relation to mental health in people with learning disabilities.

Terminology used in this book

There are many terms used to describe mental health problems, including mental illness, mental disorder, and psychiatric illness. We have adopted the term 'mental health problem(s)' to indicate that any of us can experience problems with our mental health at any time, but that does not necessarily mean that we are ill or have a disorder.

In keeping with UK policy, the term 'learning disabilities' is used throughout this book, although it is acknowledged that this does not necessarily have the same meaning internationally, and that many other terms such as developmental disability, mental retardation, and intellectual disability are in common use. Using measures of IQ as a guide, around 2% of the UK population have learning disabilities to some degree, ranging through borderline, mild, moderate, and severe to profound levels of disability (Emerson et al 2001). Where reference is made in this book to different levels of disability, this is in relation to the standard UK classification of severity of learning disability in relation to IQ, as described in DC-LD (Royal College of Psychiatrists 2001) (see Table 1). People with IQs in the range 70–80, who are often considered to have borderline learning disabilities, are likely to merge with the general population in terms of the range and manifestation of mental health problems experienced, and they are not separately considered here. However, it is important to note that learning disability should not be defined solely by performance on IQ tests, and that diagnosis now normally takes into account social and emotional factors.

Table 1 Severity of learning disability with associated IQ range (Royal College of Psychiatrists 2001)

Severity of learning disability	IQ range
Mild	50–69
Moderate	35–49
Severe	20–34
Profound	Below 20

Many terms have been used to describe the phenomenon that arises when people with learning disabilities experience mental health problems. These include the ambiguous term 'dual diagnosis' and a range of other labels. The use of labels has both advantages and disadvantages, and while this book will not dwell on these, we have struggled to find a person-friendly term to refer both to the individuals themselves and the mental health problems that they might experience. We have arrived at the somewhat wordy 'mental health problems in people with learning disabilities', and this is the term that is generally used throughout the book. For convenience, the generic term 'client' is also used frequently throughout this book, although it is acknowledged that this carries with it implications that the individual is engaged in a relationship within a professional or voluntary organisation. This should not be taken to exclude those individuals who live with their families and receive few if any interventions from outside agencies.

We use the generic terms 'carer', 'care worker', and 'care staff' somewhat interchangeably to refer to anyone who contributes in a formal or informal way to the day-to-day life of people with learning disabilities.

Finally, while much of the content of this book is relevant in an international arena, we acknowledge that most of the legislation, policy, research, and service provision referred to has a UK or even an English bias: for example, the key document *Valuing People* (Department of Health 2001) is a strategy document for England, although there are parallel documents relevant to the other UK countries such as *Fulfilling the Promises*, developed for Wales (National Assembly for Wales 2001). Material selected to illustrate key issues in this book reflects the authors' country of origin, practice, teaching and research, and should not be taken to exclude policy, legislation and practice relevant to other areas.

Helena Priest
Michael Gibbs
May 2003

REFERENCES

Bates P, Priest H, Gibbs M 2004 Education and training needs of learning disability staff in relation to mental health issues. Nurse Education in Practice (in press)

Department of Health 2001 Valuing people: a new strategy for learning disability for the 21st century. CM5086. Department of Health, London

Emerson E, Hatton C, Felce D et al 2001 Learning disabilities: the fundamental facts. Foundation for People with Learning Disabilities, London

Gibbs M, Priest H M 1999 Designing and implementing a 'dual diagnosis' module: a review of the literature and some preliminary findings. Nurse Education Today 19: 357–363

Holt G, Costello H, Oliver B 2000 Training direct care staff about the mental health needs and related issues of people with developmental disabilities. Mental Health Aspects of Developmental Disabilities 3(4): 132–139

Menolascino F J 1965 Emotional disturbance and mental retardation. American Journal of Mental Deficiency 70: 248–256

National Assembly for Wales 2001 Fulfilling the promises. What future services will look like for people with learning disabilities in Wales. National Assembly for Wales, Cardiff

Quigley A, Murray G, McKenzie K et al 2001 Staff knowledge about symptoms of mental health problems in people with learning disabilities. Journal of Learning Disabilities 5(3): 235–244

Royal College of Psychiatrists 2001 DC-LD (Diagnostic criteria for psychiatric disorders for use with adults with learning disabilities/mental retardation). Occasional Paper OP48. Gaskell, London

Abbreviations

ABC	Aberrant Behaviour Checklist
ADD	Assessment of Dual Diagnosis
BDI	Beck Depression Inventory
BILD	British Institute of Learning Disabilities
BSI	Brief Symptom Inventory
CAMHS	Child and Adolescent Mental Health Services
CAN	Camberwell Assessment of Need
CANDID	Camberwell Assessment of Need for Adults with Developmental and Intellectual Disabilities
CBT	cognitive-behaviour therapy
CPA	care programme approach
DASH-II	Diagnostic Assessment for the Severely Handicapped-II
DC-LD	Diagnostic criteria for psychiatric disorders for use with adults with learning disabilities/mental retardation
DMR	Dementia Questionnaire for Persons with Mental Retardation
EAMHMR	European Association for Mental Health in Mental Retardation
ECG	electrocardiogram
ECT	electroconvulsive therapy
GOLD	Growing Older with Learning Disabilities [programme]
GP	general practitioner
HAD	Hospital Anxiety and Depression [scale]
HIMPs	Health Improvement and Modernisation Plans
HoNOS	Health of the Nation Outcome Scales
HoNOS-LD	The Health of the Nation Outcome Scales for people with learning disabilities
HPRT	hypoxanthine-guanine phosphoribosyltransferase
IRA	individual resource allocation
JOMAAC	judgement, orientation, memory, affect, attitude, cognition
LDCNS	Learning Disabilities Version of the Cardinal Needs Schedule

MAOI	monoamine oxidase inhibitor
MAS	Motivation Assessment Scale
MMR	mumps, measles and rubella [vaccination]
MMSE	Mini-Mental State Examination
NDT	National Development Team
NHS	National Health Service
PAS-ADD	Psychiatric Assessment Schedule for Adults with Developmental Disabilities
PATH	Planning Alternative Tomorrows with Hope
PTSD	post-traumatic stress disorder
RN(LD)	registered nurse in learning disabilities
SDAT	senile dementia of the Alzheimer's type
SSRI	selective serotonin reuptake inhibitor
WHO	World Health Organization

Acknowledgements

We would like to thank all the clients, families, practitioners, colleagues, and students who have influenced the conceptualisation of this book, and who have so generously contributed experiences and ideas that have influenced its content and organisation.

Thanks also go to Catherine Jackson at Elsevier for keeping us on track.

Finally, we are indebted to our families and friends, and in particular to John and Sue, without whose support and encouragement the book would not have materialised.

Helena Priest
Michael Gibbs
May 2003

The mental health needs of people with learning disabilities: background and context

INTRODUCTION

In this chapter we will introduce both learning disabilities and mental health problems, initially from a historical perspective, in order to provide a background and context for discussion of contemporary perspectives and approaches. The concept of mental health in relation to people with learning disabilities will be explored and epidemiological and research data presented to compare the occurrence and frequency of mental health problems in people with learning disabilities with the general population. Relevant terms will be defined, and finally, the role of carers working with this client group will be explored.

We begin by introducing Geoff, a man with learning disabilities who may have mental health problems. As you read the rest of this chapter, you may like to reflect on whether what you are reading helps you to understand his unique situation, and whether it helps you to begin to see how you might respond to his needs.

Case study: Geoff

Geoff is a 56-year-old man who lives in a house with four other men who have all recently left a local hospital for people with learning disabilities. Geoff had been a resident in the hospital for 40 years, but the hospital has recently closed. He has moderate learning disabilities and takes an active part in the day-to-day running of the home, including carrying out domestic activities with the help of his key worker. His verbal skills are limited but he has a good command of Makaton (a non-verbal communication system using signs and pictures). Normally, Geoff is good natured and easy going, but he is occasionally verbally aggressive towards one of the other residents. When new staff are introduced to the home he likes to spend time showing them photographs of holidays and his collection of paintings that he completed on an art course at the hospital's Occupational Therapy department.

As Geoff's key worker in the house, you have noticed that his general appearance has changed recently, and that he is no longer following his usual routine of washing and keeping his room tidy. Other staff have reported that he sometimes shouts out for no obvious reason. Occasionally he gets up in the early hours of the morning and wanders around the house, which is causing other people living in the house to complain to the staff.

We will return to Geoff's story throughout this chapter, but first we will turn our attention to the nature of learning disability itself.

WHAT IS LEARNING DISABILITY?

Learning disability, as defined in the UK, is a state of impaired intelligence and social functioning, which started before adulthood, and which has a lasting effect on development (Department of Health 2001). Learning disability can develop in the womb, for example as a result of genetic defects, metabolic disorders, or infections; it can occur as a result of difficulties during childbirth resulting in lack of oxygen to the brain; or it can be the result of an injury to the brain in childhood. The term 'learning disability' itself can be confusing. In the USA, it means a disorder of the basic processes involved in understanding or using language, such as dyslexia, or in doing mathematical calculations. Currently it is acceptable internationally to use the terms 'mental retardation', 'intellectual disability', or 'developmental disability', but other terms such as 'mental handicap', 'mental subnormality', and 'learning difficulty' have been used in the past, and are still used in some contexts today. However, in the UK the Department of Health (1992) adopted the term 'learning disabilities' to identify those people with an IQ below 70 (IQ stands for intelligence quotient, as measured by an intelligence test), and it is this term that will predominantly be used throughout this book.

History of learning disabilities – attitudes, beliefs and responses

The idea that people with learning disabilities can, and do, experience mental health problems has only recently begun to receive significant attention, although the possibility was first recorded in the mid-19th century and given serious attention by Menolascino in 1965. In order to understand why and how people with learning disabilities might experience mental health problems, it is important to explore the ways in which they have lived and been perceived and treated by others in the past. Early accounts of learning disabilities argued that if someone was born an 'idiot' (a label in use for many years, right up until the early part of the 20th century), then this was as a result of evil doing or was a punishment for sin. Other accounts suggested that people with learning disabilities were non-humans, brought to earth by elves and fairies (Ryan & Thomas 1987). By the 14th century a distinction was made between 'idiots' (people with learning disabilities) and 'lunatics' (people with mental health problems) for the purpose of deciding whether or not to allow them to inherit property. If a man had lost his power of reason due to lunacy or madness, it was assumed that his reason could be regained, and therefore he could inherit property; whereas those born as idiots were believed not to have any understanding, therefore their property would be given to the king, who assumed all rights over them (O'Conner & Tizard 1956). By the 17th century legal definitions were produced determining different levels of learning disability, and by the late 1700s a clear distinction had been made between insanity and learning disability. At this time, also, the view that learning disability was incurable was confirmed. Early records from the mid to late 1800s show that although there were clear distinctions, which led to the development of legal definitions, there was still uncertainty in the relationship between learning disability and mental health problems, and both client groups were typically cared for within the same institutions.

During the early 1800s there was a determined effort to help people with mental disorders, regardless of whether these originated from learning disabilities or other mental health problems. In Europe, in particular, some influential services were developed. When Pinel, a French doctor, became responsible for mental health facilities in Paris he found the living conditions and treatment approaches to be unacceptable. Hence he developed programmes of care that focused on the environment, social activities, and moral management rather than former oppressive approaches that included abuse, chaining, and other degrading practices. Similarly, in Britain, William Tuke developed a humane regime of care at the Retreat, an institution in York. In 1801, Itard published *The Wild Boy of Aveyron*, a study of work carried out with Victor, a young boy who was found living wild in the forests outside Paris. Itard adopted training methods based on reinforcement and reward to encourage Victor's development. At the time, many reports suggested that Itard could not succeed, as it was believed that a person who was delayed in development could not improve. Hence, Itard was led to believe that he had failed in his efforts with Victor; nonetheless in time he became recognised as one of the founders of modern special education. Seguin, his student, developed Itard's work further, and became the first person to develop an educational service for people with learning disabilities in France; he also travelled to North America and developed educational services there. After the publication of Itard's work several others followed, such as Guggenbahl in Switzerland and Reed in England, both of whom established residential educational services for people with learning disabilities, with the primary aim of educating pupils to a level that would allow them to return to society as productive members.

By the latter half of the 1800s, in parts of Europe, state education for children with learning disabilities was compulsory. It seemed, then, that in the 1800s the care and education available for people with learning disabilities had become somewhat more humane in its approach.

However, subsequent changes in society began to reverse that positive trend. Firstly, increasing industrialisation highlighted the fact that there were many people with learning disabilities who lacked the necessary skills to enable them to contribute effectively to the developing industrial working environments and practices, whereas they may have functioned adequately in former agriculturally dominated times. This led to them being rejected as invalid members of society, and fostered a desire for them to be removed from it. These actions were justified by the eugenics movement. The term 'eugenics' was first used in the late 1800s and was defined by Galton in 1883 as 'the science of improving inborn human qualities through selective breeding' (Atherton 2003). The eugenics movement gathered apace during the industrial revolution, when people were judged by their ability to deal with new demands in relation to changing industrial practices. People with learning disabilities could now be identified as one group of people that could not adjust to these changes, and thus they came to be seen as a burden on society. Strong beliefs in the eugenics principles led to segregation and social stigma towards them. They came to be seen as 'feeble-minded', and, as the general public became better educated and better informed, a sense of moral panic ensued. Thus the attitudes of society had changed from those of a philanthropic nature to those that urged a more custodial and segregated system of care provision. It is not difficult to imagine that these negative attitudes and exclusion practices would have had a devastating impact on the emotions and self-esteem of people with learning disabilities.

The second change, in response to these attitudes, was the rapid growth of institutional care during the latter half of the 19th and the first half of the 20th century, manifested by the building of many large mental deficiency 'colonies', which gradually reversed enlightened care regimes. If, for example, families had children with learning disabilities, they were now encouraged to put them into an institution rather than to have them educated. Adults with learning disabilities were admitted into institutions as an effective means of removing them from the sight and conscience of the general population. In part due to overcrowding and negative staff attitudes, and in part due to changes in societal values, institutions changed from promoting humanistic and environmental approaches based on moral values to medically and scientifically dominated approaches, in which people with learning disabilities became 'inmates' and eventually, with the advent of the National Health Service in 1948, 'patients'. These changes were not necessarily in the best interests of people with learning disabilities and, as we shall see, may have contributed to the development of mental health problems.

Institutional life was soon shown to have devastating adverse effects on individual lives. Goffman (1968), in his classic work *Asylums*, studied these negative effects of institutional care, brought about by batch living, whereby all patients lived, slept, worked and played in the same establishment according to the same routines, thereby losing any sense of individuality, identity, and control. Barton (1959) highlighted the negative effects further through the concept of 'institutional neurosis'. Through his work he showed that institutional care created a disease process in its own right. This disease was characterised by apathy, lack of initiative, loss of interest, submissiveness, lack of individuality, and sometimes a characteristic stooping and shuffling posture and gait. Patients were largely browbeaten into conforming to routines by staff attitudes. Although Barton's observations were made within mental health institutions, he argued that these effects could occur in any institution. It could be surmised, then, that these effects would be experienced by people with learning disabilities living in institutions, demonstrating the potential for mental health problems to occur in people with learning disabilities.

While institutions created institutionalisation for some people, for others disturbed behaviours such as self-injury and aggression were the consequence (Stenfert Kroese & Holmes 2001). These authors further postulated that people with learning disabilities in institutions were sometimes at the mercy of experimental medication and behavioural treatments, or interventions based on punishment and isolation. Furthermore, they were often devalued through being obliged to carry out menial and sometimes meaningless tasks in the name of 'occupation'.

Hence, although institutions theoretically provided security, treatment and care, it soon became clear that they were not, after all, places of safety, and were more likely to cause problems, including mental health problems, for people with learning disabilities than to solve them. As succinctly summarised by Beacock (2003, p 54):

What has clearly happened is that a vulnerable group of people has been subjected to a system of care and a lifestyle that has promoted the development of a secondary diagnosis of mental illness in many.

Before we examine the more recent history of learning disabilities it may be useful to reflect on some of the issues identified so far.

Exercise
Reflect on the historical accounts of attitudes, care and treatment for people with learning disabilities, and try to explain how and why these have changed in the present day.

You are likely to have concluded that, in the more distant past, members of society who were in some way 'different' from the norm were included within their community, but as industrial society and education developed, so too did more negative attitudes and values. People who were obviously 'different' due to their appearance and level of ability attracted negative attitudes to the extent that they became seen as defects of society and became excluded from it. The language used to describe the client group reflected these negative values, with labels such as 'idiot', 'moron', and 'moral defective' commonly applied.

Today, things are very different. Systems of care are based on valuing the social role of each individual with learning disabilities, rooted in the normalisation principles of the 1950s and beyond, and more recently in the principles and policies of person centred planning, rights, inclusion, and community care (Department of Health 2001). The 1960s heralded these developments, with changes both in the administration of care and in its underpinning philosophical approach. The Mental Health Act of 1959 established the principle of community care, and, although this was not an entirely new concept, the Act made it clear how community care was to be implemented. The decision to move from institutional care to community care for people with learning disabilities produced a vision of changing that care from a medical, hospital-based, biological model to a social, community, environmental model, thus also bringing into question the nature of learning disability itself. In the institutional, medical mode, learning disabilities were seen as the responsibility of scientists, doctors, and nurses, who could initiate scientific research and take care of their patients' physiological and health needs. In the social mode, however, learning disabilities became viewed in a much more complex way. Clients were no longer necessarily considered ill, and therefore would not necessarily need the skills of doctors and nurses.

Equally, the language that is used today to describe clients has changed to embrace more acceptable and less stigmatising labels including the current 'learning disabilities' or 'developmental disabilities'. Labelling can contribute to stigma and low self-worth; hence the use of less negative terms should contribute towards the improvement in clients' self-perceptions and self-esteem.

What might be concluded, then, is that improvements in attitudes, and in corresponding care practices, have improved the life of people with learning disabilities, to the extent that at least some of the factors contributing to the development of mental health problems should have been eradicated. But was this really the case? This question will be addressed later in this chapter. Before that, however, the nature of mental health problems will be explored.

MENTAL HEALTH PROBLEMS

According to the American Psychiatric Association (1994, p xxi), a mental health problem, or mental disorder, is:

...a clinically significant behavioral or psychological syndrome or pattern...that is associated with present distress or disability or with a significantly increased risk of suffering, death, pain, disability, or an important loss of freedom.

Put more simply, a mental health problem can be said to exist when there is a change in an individual's mood, behaviour, and thought processes to such an extent that day-to-day life, activities, and relationships are adversely affected. No-one is born with a mental health problem and, in many cases, mental health problems will resolve themselves with or without intervention from health care professionals. In Chapter 2, we will consider in greater depth some of the theories that are available today to explain why mental health problems occur, but, put very simply, mental health problems normally arise out of a combination of:

- predisposing physical or biological factors
- factors that increase a person's vulnerability, such as adverse childhood experiences, poor coping strategies, or lack of support
- external stressful events.

Often, a person can cope perfectly well with a huge number of difficulties, but may reach the point where a new difficulty, even if minor, becomes 'the last straw that breaks the camel's back'.

MENTAL HEALTH PROBLEMS AND PEOPLE WITH LEARNING DISABILITIES

When people with learning disabilities experience a mental health problem, they are sometimes referred to as having a dual diagnosis, which means the coexistence of two conditions – in this case, learning disabilities and a mental health problem. The term 'dual diagnosis' can be misleading, as it is used in many other health contexts. It is frequently used, for example, to describe substance misuse coexisting with a mental health problem. Although wordy, the phrase 'mental health problems in people with learning disabilities' is a more accurate descriptor. The coexistence of learning disabilities and mental health problems has been acknowledged for some time, and yet it has only recently become the centre of attention due to changes in philosophical approaches to care and attitudes and beliefs about people with learning disabilities. This new awareness has been heightened by the move from institutional to community care, prior to which little attention was paid to the mental health needs of people with learning disabilities. As we have seen, life inside a long stay hospital, or institution, was thought to be one of the causes of mental health problems. Hence it was believed that the closure of these hospitals would help to eliminate such problems. With the move towards community care, and a care regime based on rights, values, and choice, it was envisaged that mental health problems would reduce. However, it now seems that the move to community care may actually have increased the likelihood of mental health problems occurring. As people with learning disabilities move to community settings they become exposed to greater demands (Emerson & Hatton 1994). They are faced with stress factors such as bereavement caused by staff or friendship changes, moving home and other new life events, and yet they may not have developed adequate coping strategies to deal with these challenges. Some are facing complexities of life never previously experienced. At the same time, they are being faced with new risks, challenges, and decisions. These experiences could be contributory factors in the incidence of stress, depression, and other forms of mental health problems.

The extent of the problem

Why are the mental health needs of people with learning disabilities only now receiving attention? One explanation is that, in the past, people with learning disabilities were thought to be incapable of experiencing mental health problems, due to their cognitive and intellectual deficits. Any observed changes in mood and behaviour would therefore have been interpreted and explained as part of their learning disability, a concept described as *diagnostic overshadowing* by Reiss et al (1982; for a fuller discussion of diagnostic overshadowing, see Ch. 3). An alternative explanation (Szymanski & Grossman 1984) is that the emotional states of people with learning disabilities are qualitatively different from those of the general population, and that these emotional states are of biological origin. However, it is now generally agreed that people with learning disabilities can and do experience mental health problems. Indeed, prevalence rates are generally agreed to be higher in the learning disabled population than in the general population (Došen & Day 2001).

This finding applies to all levels of disability and all age groups, and is a universally observed phenomenon. In the UK, for example, Birch et al (1970) suggested that prevalence rates in adults were over 40% in people with severe learning disabilities compared with 10% in those in the non-learning disabled population. Tonge et al (1996) found a similar rate in Australia. Higher prevalence rates are seen across different age groups; for example, Strømme & Diseth (2000), in a study of children in Norway, found a prevalence rate of 33% in children with mild learning disabilities, rising to 42% in children with severe learning disabilities. Borthwick-Duffy (1994) reviewed 12 epidemiological studies of children and adolescents and found a range from less than 10% to 80%, with an average of 45%. In a British study of over 10 000 young people aged 5–15 years, Emerson (2003) concluded that young people with learning disabilities are at a significantly higher risk of certain forms of mental health problems, including anxiety and pervasive developmental disorders, compared with non-learning disabled people of the same age. Literature regarding mental health problems in the older learning disabled population is more limited; however, Sansom et al (1994) found that 12.9% of 124 hospital residents with learning disabilities aged between 60 and 94 had a diagnosis of dementia, 8.9% had a diagnosis of affective disorder, and 6.5% had a diagnosis of schizophrenia.

There is now general consensus that around 40% of people using learning disability services have additional mental health needs (Emerson et al 2001). Furthermore, although there is limited research evidence in relation to diagnosis, prevalence and treatment (Hatton 2002), it appears that for almost all common mental health problems, prevalence is significantly higher in people with learning disabilities than in the non-learning disabled population (Borthwick-Duffy 1994, Crews et al 1994). In particular, there is evidence to support high rates of psychosis, notably schizophrenia, in people with learning disabilities (Došen & Day 2001, Hatton 2002), and high rates of depression and dementia in people with Down's syndrome (Hatton 2002).

Anxiety is reported as being at least as common in people with mild learning disabilities as in the general population, and dysthymia (an enduring and prolonged depressed mood) is said to be more common (Došen & Day 2001). The evidence relating to depression is somewhat conflicting, with some studies reporting rates as high as 40% and yet others reporting rates for major depression as being similar to the general population, around 1–2%. These differences may be due to the level of learning disability and the severity of the depression in the populations studied, or to the ways in which data are gathered. Despite this sometimes conflicting evidence, it seems that the existence of mental health problems generally is a major concern for those involved with people with learning disabilities.

Exercise
Why do you think that estimates of prevalence vary so much?

There are many problems in trying to establish the prevalence of mental health problems in people with learning disabilities. These problems stem from two main factors: definitional and identification issues, and data collection methods.

Definitional and identification issues

There is a range of definitions of learning disabilities, including IQ, that give a numerical label, together with social, educational and psychological definitions, all of which can blur the parameters of what learning disabilities actually are. Furthermore, there is conflicting evidence in relation to whether mental health problems are more or less common in people with severe learning disabilities than in those with mild learning disabilities (Deb et al 2001). It is possible, therefore, that cases of mental health problems at either end of the ability spectrum may have been overlooked.

Some prevalence studies include personality disorder, autism, attention deficit hyperactivity disorder, and dementia as examples of mental health problems, while others do not (Deb et al 2001). Another reason for the variance in prevalence rates is related to challenging behaviours. If challenging behaviours are considered to be manifestations of mental health problems, then prevalence rates will be higher than if these behaviours are interpreted as part of the learning disability itself. We will discuss challenging behaviour in greater depth in Chapter 3.

Data collection methods

A second difficulty in identifying prevalence rates is that they vary depending on the methods used to collect data. Many studies have relied upon institutional rather than community populations, thus neglecting the possibility of mental health problems occurring in people with learning disabilities living independently in their own homes or with families, and many are based on retrospective data from cases notes rather than observations and direct patient interviews. These factors may have contributed to sampling bias (Deb et al 2001).

Other prevalence factors

Sovner (1986) has provided further explanations that might account for such variation in prevalence rates. He describes a range of barriers that influence how mental health problems are presented and interpreted in people with learning disabilities. These include intellectual distortion and psychological masking.

- *Intellectual distortion* occurs when a low level of skills and functioning of people with learning disabilities leads to a difficulty in their expressing or communicating internal feelings. As assessment and diagnosis rely so heavily on the client's communication ability, then if the client is unable to communicate emotions effectively there is a chance that any mental health problems will be overlooked, and appropriate care and services will not be received.
- *Psychological masking* occurs when the client's life experience has been limited compared with the general population; thus mental health symptoms do not appear to be as significant as they might in a person without learning disabilities.

These barriers, and others, are discussed in more detail in Chapter 3, but already we are beginning to see the difficulties in accurately identifying the existence of mental health problems in people with learning disabilities.

THE ROLE OF CARERS

Many people with learning disabilities lead a relatively independent life, but others require some sort of assistance, either from their families, or from health or social care services. Today there is an ongoing debate about how people with learning disabilities who also have a mental health problem should be treated, and which services should provide care and treatment. It is argued, on the one hand, that, in the spirit of social inclusion, community presence and participation (Department of Health 2001), they should receive care from mainstream mental health services. The advantage of this is that people with learning disabilities will be valued and treated exactly the same as any other user of mental health services, and will have access to a wealth of expertise in mental health assessment and intervention. On the other hand, it can be argued that mainstream mental health services are not routinely designed to cater for people with learning disabilities, and therefore may not adequately understand and respond to their unique needs; hence care and support should come from specialists in the field. In this book, we will argue that people with learning disabilities do have needs that are not necessarily the same as those of non-learning disabled people, and that the services they need may not always be available in the mainstream sector. A more detailed discussion of services, and examples of good practice, can be found in Chapter 9.

For those people who need support and care from health or social services, it is staff members working in these services that they will rely upon to recognise changes in their mental health state. One of the skills required is to be able to draw out the issues in a person's life that can lead to a comprehensive assessment of mental health state. This is not easy, as although the presentation of mental health problems in people with mild learning disabilities may be similar to that in the general population, it is much more difficult to identify problems in clients with moderate or severe learning disabilities.

Unfortunately, it seems that many carers are limited in their understanding of mental health care needs, and are sometimes lacking in the skills and resources required to assess needs and deliver appropriate care (Bates et al 2004, Gibbs & Priest 1999, Holt et al 2000, Quigley et al 2001). This is one of the reasons why this book has been written. While many professionals and carers are highly educated and trained, often in specialist interventions such as cognitive–behavioural therapy, group psychotherapy, drama, music and art therapy, there has until recently been a lack of educational provision for people working in learning disability settings wishing to develop their knowledge, understanding and skill in the field of mental health as it relates to their client group. This deficit is currently being addressed in the UK by, for example, the provision of university courses leading to recognised qualifications, together with a range of shorter study days, conferences, and training programmes, such as those organised by the National Development Team (NDT) and the British Institute of Learning Disabilities (BILD). It is hoped that these will continue to help staff to develop the knowledge and skills that will be of greatest benefit to the client group.

CASE STUDY REFLECTIONS

At the beginning of this chapter, we introduced Geoff, and suggested that you might reflect on his story as you read the chapter. Having done so, you may have identified some of the following issues that are relevant to his life and current experiences.

Firstly, Geoff has spent many years in institutional care. Although this may have been a positive experience for him, in that it provided total care, security, routine, and occupation, he may have experienced some of the negative effects of institutional living such as apathy, submissiveness, lack of individuality, and lack of control over his daily activities. If so, we might expect that now he has left the institution, he will have a better quality of life, with greater control over his lifestyle, greater privacy, more individual attention, better access to community facilities and activities, and that his unique personality will now be afforded greater recognition.

However, we must consider what Geoff has lost in this major change to his life. He may no longer be living with familiar people, and the staff in the house may be different from those he knew in the hospital. Hence his previous social network and familiar sources of support may no longer be available to him. He may in fact have less freedom than in the institutional setting, which typically would have had extensive gardens and open spaces. As Geoff has limited verbal communication skills, he may have difficulties in expressing his emotional needs, and hence the chances of carers failing to identify such needs are high. Furthermore, it may be that in the climate of person centred planning, Geoff is experiencing pressure to make choices and take decisions in aspects of his life over which he previously had little control and few responsibilities.

Research reviewed by Emerson & Hatton (1994) on the effects of relocating from hospital to community showed that although clients could expect a better standard of living, more contacts with other people, more support from staff, more opportunities for choice, and greater use of community facilities, they do in fact have few opportunities to exercise choice, few relationships within the community, little presence in the community, little contact from staff, and rarely develop new skills. Some or all of these factors may have contributed to Geoff's current emotional state and behaviour.

However, on a positive note, it has been concluded that small group living offers a better quality of life for people with learning disabilities than either institutional or large community provision. The challenge then is for staff within such small group living settings to help clients to maximise their physical, emotional and social well-being with the hope of preventing or minimising the effects of mental health problems occurring in the future.

CONCLUSION

This chapter has introduced many of the challenges faced by practitioners in the field of learning disabilities in addressing their clients' mental health needs. Starting with a historical overview, it has identified a number of issues that need to be addressed in order for this client group to receive the appropriate care that they require to live as full a life as possible. The fact that this client group do have mental health needs is clear, but exactly how many have mental health problems, and the exact nature of those problems, is more difficult to quantify. The role of carers is vital, whether they are professionally qualified, unqualified, or family members or friends, and these people need adequate support to help maintain the mental health status of their clients. The remaining chapters of this book are intended to help the reader to answer some of the as yet unanswered questions, and discuss the key issues. In Chapter 2 we will begin to explore in more detail some of the theories and explanations about mental health problems in people with learning disabilities.

REFERENCES

American Psychiatric Association 1994 Diagnostic and statistical manual of mental disorders DSM-IV, 4th edn. American Psychiatric Association, Washington
Atherton H 2003 A history of learning disabilities. In: Gates B (ed) Learning disabilities: towards inclusion, 4th edn. Churchill Livingstone, Edinburgh, p 41–60
Barton R 1959 Institutional neurosis, 2nd edn. Wright, Bristol
Bates P, Priest H, Gibbs M 2004 Education and training needs of learning disability staff in relation to mental health issues. Nurse Education in Practice (in press)
Beacock C 2003 Mental health in learning disabilities. In: Marwick A, Parish A (eds) Learning disabilities: themes and perspectives. Butterworth Heinemann, Oxford, p 43–63
Birch H, Richardson S, Baird D et al 1970 Mental subnormality in the community: a clinical and epidemiological study. Williams and Wilkins, Baltimore
Borthwick-Duffy S A 1994 Epidemiology and prevalence of psychopathology in people with mental retardation. Journal of Consulting and Clinical Psychology 62: 17–27
Crews D W, Bonaventura S, Rowe F 1994 Dual diagnosis: prevalence of psychiatric disorders in a large state residential facility for individuals with mental retardation. American Journal on Mental Retardation 98(6): 688–731
Deb S, Matthews T, Holt G et al 2001 Practice guidelines for the assessment and diagnosis of mental health problems in adults with intellectual disability. Pavilion, Brighton
Department of Health 1992 Social care for adults with learning disabilities (mental handicap). LAC (92)15. HMSO, London
Department of Health 2001 Valuing people: a new strategy for learning disability for the 21st century. CM5086. Department of Health, London
Došen A, Day K 2001 Treating mental illness and behaviour disorders in children and adults with mental retardation. American Psychiatric Press, Washington
Emerson E 2003 Prevalence of psychiatric disorders in children and adolescents with and without intellectual disability. Journal of Intellectual Disability Research 47(1): 51–58

Emerson E, Hatton C 1994 Moving out: relocation from hospital to community. HMSO, London

Emerson E, Hatton C, Felce D et al 2001 Learning disabilities: the fundamental facts. The Mental Health Foundation, London

Gibbs M, Priest H M 1999 Designing and implementing a 'dual diagnosis' module: a review of the literature and some preliminary findings. Nurse Education Today 19: 357–363

Goffman E 1968 Asylums. Essays on the social situation of mental patients and other inmates. Penguin, Harmondsworth

Hatton C 2002 Psychosocial interventions for adults with intellectual disabilities and mental health problems: a review. Journal of Mental Health 11(4): 357–373

Holt G, Costello H, Oliver B 2000 Training direct care staff about the mental health needs and related issues of people with developmental disabilities. Mental Health Aspects of Developmental Disabilities 3(4): 132–139

Menolascino F J 1965 Emotional disturbance and mental retardation. American Journal of Mental Deficiency 70: 248–256

O'Conner N, Tizard J 1956 The social problem of mental deficiency. Pergamon, London

Quigley A, Murray G, McKenzie K et al 2001 Staff knowledge about symptoms of mental health problems in people with learning disabilities. Journal of Learning Disabilities 5(3): 235–244

Reiss S, Levitan G, Szyszko J 1982 Emotional disturbance and mental retardation: diagnostic overshadowing. American Journal of Mental Deficiency 86: 567–574

Ryan J, Thomas F 1987 The politics of mental handicap. Free Association Books, London

Sansom D T, Singh I, Jawed S H 1994 Elderly people with learning disabilities in hospital: a psychiatric study. Journal of Intellectual Disability Research 38: 287–294

Sovner R 1986 Limiting factors in the use of DSM-III criteria with mentally ill/mentally retarded persons. Psychopharmacology Bulletin 24(4): 1055–1059

Stenfert Kroese B, Holmes G 2001 'I've never said "no" to anything in my life': helping people with learning disabilities who experience psychological problems. In: Newnes C, Holmes G, Dunn C (eds) This is madness too. Critical perspectives on mental health services. PCCS Books, Llangarron, p 71–80

Strømme P, Diseth T H 2000 Prevalence of psychiatric diagnoses in children with mental retardation: data from a population-based study. Developmental Medicine and Child Neurology 42: 266–270

Szymanski L S, Grossman H 1984 Dual implications of 'dual diagnosis'. Mental Retardation 22: 155–156

Tonge B, Einfeld S, Krupinski J et al 1996 The use of factor analysis for ascertaining patterns of psychopathology in children with intellectual disability. Journal of Intellectual Disability Research 40: 198–207

2

Explaining the problem

INTRODUCTION

In Chapter 1, we began to explore the nature of mental health problems, and some of the reasons why people with learning disabilities might be at particular risk of developing mental health problems. In this chapter, we will review in greater depth a number of explanations for the occurrence of mental health problems, both in the general population and, specifically, in relation to people with learning disabilities. Based on holistic principles, the chapter will discuss biological, psychological, and social explanations, and consider ways in which explanations are sometimes combined through the concept of eclecticism. The chapter will, in addition, discuss a range of vulnerability factors that might predispose people with learning disabilities to develop mental health problems. Therapeutic interventions arising from the various explanations of mental health problems will be introduced, although these will be explored more thoroughly in Chapter 7.

In this chapter, we introduce Jason, a young man with learning disabilities who seems to be developing some problems that are causing concern to his family and friends. As you read the chapter, try to identify possible reasons why he might be experiencing these difficulties in his life.

Case study: Jason

Jason is a 16-year-old boy with mild learning disabilities. He lives at home with his mother and attends the local comprehensive school, where he has a Statement of Special Educational Needs, and is supported in his lessons by a member of the learning support staff. His IQ has been measured as 65. His parents are divorced and he no longer has contact with his father, but he knows that his father had a 'nervous breakdown' some years ago. He is shortly to sit some end of year examinations and after that he will leave his present school. He is uncertain about whether or where he will continue his education. Jason has always been a keen athlete and is a member of the local junior football club. He has a wide circle of friends, and together they spend evenings at the local youth club, at the swimming baths, or watching videos at each other's houses.

Until a few weeks ago Jason had a Saturday job at the local supermarket, where he collected trolleys and ran errands. However, he recently lost this job as he had become unreliable, turning up late and scruffy in appearance. Staff complained that he would often appear to be daydreaming and not responding to their requests or instructions. Jason did not seem to be particularly upset at losing his job, and he now spends most of his Saturdays in bed or in his room staring out of the window. On several occasions, when his friends have called for him to go out, he has asked his mum to tell them he is not feeling well. His mum is concerned and has asked the GP for advice.

Exercise

Imagine that you are a professional community worker who has been asked to visit Jason and his mother to make an assessment of their needs and problems.

- What do you think might be happening?
- What might have caused the recent changes in Jason's behaviour?

As you may have discovered, the questions about Jason have no simple answers:

- Could it be that his problems are due to loss of contact with his father?
- Does the fact that his father had a 'nervous breakdown' some time ago offer us any clues?
- Could it be that Jason is under pressure due to worry about his exams, or about having to make choices about further education or employment?
- Why has he become reluctant to socialise? Are there some difficulties in his relationships with his friends?
- Could all of these factors be relevant in trying to understand Jason's recent change in mood and behaviour? Or none of them?
- Might he have a mental health problem, or can we explain the changes in his behaviour in another way?

As we shall see, explanations for the onset of mental health problems are rarely clear-cut. To some extent, early theories about what might cause mental health problems have been derived from developments in treatment approaches in psychiatry. For example, in the 1950s, drugs were developed to address the symptoms of schizophrenia, and electroconvulsive therapy was found to be effective in treating severe depression. Thus, the finding that mental health problems could be controlled by physiological or chemical means lent support to the theory that mental health problems had physiological origins. In the 1960s, the successful use of behaviour modification systems to teach clients to adapt behaviours to be within more acceptable limits lent weight to the theory that mental health and behavioural problems were caused by faulty learning, and could be corrected by appropriate relearning processes. We will explore these and other theories in this chapter, but will commence with an overview of the history of beliefs and ideas about the causation of mental health problems, before moving on to consider contemporary explanations, and their relevance for people with learning disabilities today.

HISTORY OF MENTAL HEALTH BELIEFS AND TREATMENT APPROACHES

Mental health problems have been recognised for thousands of years, and there has long been a desire to understand and explain the origins of these problems. As with the history of learning disability, outlined in Chapter 1, explanations have, in the main, been consistent with society's prevailing norms, beliefs, and state of knowledge, and many early attempts to define and explain mental health problems have long fallen out of general acceptance. Nonetheless, the many and varied explanations proposed over the centuries have contributed to current knowledge. Consequently, there exists today a range of models that aim both to explain the cause of a particular mental health problem and to treat it appropriately.

From the second century AD, right through the Middle Ages and into the beginning of the 19th century, supernatural beliefs often led to mental disorders being explained as possession by demons or evil spirits. Consequently, treatments were aimed at the removal of these spirits from the body, often by physical means such as whipping, ducking in water, bleeding, and purging. During the 16th century, mass burnings were common, but by the 17th century the move to mass containment within institutions or asylums had begun. During the 18th century, in parallel with attitudes towards people with learning disabilities, there was something of a change in thinking; patients were less likely to be seen as evil, and treatment approaches became somewhat more humane. However, by the 19th and early 20th century, which, as we have seen, saw massive expansion in the provision of institutions, mental health problems had become firmly medicalised, in concordance with rapid developments in scientific and medical knowledge. Symptoms were most likely to be explained as the result of physical illness, and consequently the dominant explanation of the nature and causation of mental health problems became the biological or disease model. To some extent, this remains the case today, particularly in psychiatry as it is practised within the UK National Health Service (NHS), not least because all psychiatrists are medically qualified before specialising in psychiatry.

Biological or disease model

Originating from the time of Hippocrates, the father of modern medicine, this model explains mental health problems as a consequence of physical and/or chemical changes in the body, particularly in the brain and nervous system. Furthermore, genetic factors may cause or predispose individuals to specific biochemical changes. Much modern psychiatry reflects this perspective, and systematic examination of patients for the presence or absence of mental disorder takes the same approach as for physical disease. A psychiatric diagnosis is normally made according to a formal classification system such as ICD-10 (World Health Organization 1992) or DSM-IV (American Psychiatric Association 1994, 2000), and treatment methods are aimed at altering brain function without harming healthy parts of the patient's body or functioning. Thus it follows that treatment will use physical or chemical means to reverse the problem or prevent further deterioration. If, for example, it can be shown that symptoms or behaviours are related to brain chemistry, then the application of chemicals in the form of medication might be the treatment approach of choice. Physical treatments include electroconvulsive therapy and psychosurgery, although the latter is little used today (see Ch. 7 for more discussion of these treatments).

Before proceeding to explore other explanations of mental health problems, a word of caution in relation to the biological or disease model is appropriate here. While it is well accepted that there are associations between many forms of mental health problem and physical or chemical changes in the body, with very few exceptions it cannot be assumed that these changes actually *cause* the problem. It is likely that many more years of research will be necessary to demonstrate direct causal relationships between brain structure and function and a whole range of mental health problems. For example, many studies have identified abnormalities in the brains of people with schizophrenia (see Ch. 4). However, at this time it is not possible to say that these abnormalities actually *cause* schizophrenia; indeed, they may prove to be an *effect* of schizophrenia. Furthermore, it would be difficult to separate the effects of brain structure and function from other factors, such as environment, infection, or family stress, which may contribute to the onset of schizophrenia. As a further example, although changes in the brains of people with Alzheimer's disease (see Ch. 4) can clearly be identified at post-mortem examination, it is not entirely clear what causes these changes, and why some people experience them and others do not.

Having explored the contribution of the medical or disease model to our understanding of mental health problems, let us now turn to explore a range of psychological explanations.

Psychological models

A psychological model seeks to identify not a physical or biological explanation for mental health problems, but rather to look for explanations within the person's childhood development and experience, learning experiences, environment, self-concept, thoughts and feelings. Four major psychological explanations exist: the psychodynamic model, the behavioural model, the cognitive model, and the humanistic model. All, with the exception of the behavioural model, explain mental health problems as rooted within the individual rather than being external to the individual. We will look at each of these in turn.

Psychodynamic model

This model has its origins in late 19th and early 20th century, the major exponents being Freud (1856–1939), Jung (1875–1961), and Adler (1870–1937). The notion of the unconscious is central to this model, i.e. the belief that mental activity takes place outside the individual's conscious awareness, yet influences behaviour, and may produce 'symptoms'. Symptoms may be the result of conflict between creative and destructive forces within the unconscious, and may have their roots in early childhood experiences and relationships. The individual may not be aware of these inner conflicts, due to the operation of defence mechanisms such as repression or denial, which serve to reduce anxiety. For example, someone who has experienced major trauma or abuse in childhood may unconsciously bury all memories of that experience so that the unpleasant memories do not have to be faced and dealt with in adult life. However, when defence mechanisms fail to be effective, the person is likely to experience conflict, anxiety, or depression. Freud, together with Erikson (1902–1994) suggested that the life course follows a series of stages, each of which has to be successfully completed before progressing to the next stage of psychological development. If not, the individual will take forward unresolved problems and conflicts that are likely to affect their mental health adversely in later life.

Psychodynamic treatment methods are directed towards the underlying problem rather than the symptoms, with the aim of resolving unconscious conflict, and include 'talking therapies' such as individual or group psychotherapy, and some forms of creative therapies such as art therapy or psychodrama (see Ch. 7 for further discussion on these therapies).

Behavioural model

This model has a long history of use both as an explanatory device and as a treatment modality in mental health and learning disability care. It has its origins in the early 20th century, and is based on the theories of learning arising out of the experimental work of Pavlov (1849–1936) and Skinner (1904–1990). It proposes that all behaviour occurs as a result of learning, and that environmental factors influence this behaviour. Thus, undesirable symptoms or behaviours are seen as habits acquired through maladaptive learning processes. In other words, the symptoms *are* the problem; therefore, removing the symptoms through a relearning process should solve the problem. Thus, treatment approaches focus on altering observable behaviours. They include *behaviour therapy*, based on the work of Pavlov, which aims to replace faulty learned associations with alternative, desirable ones; and *behaviour modification*, based on the work of Skinner, which aims to change behaviour by manipulating the consequences of behaviour such as rewards or punishment. In practice, the term 'behaviour therapy' is often used to describe any intervention designed to change or modify behaviour.

Social learning theory, first proposed by Albert Bandura (1925–), is an extension of these early theories of learning and behaviour. It suggests that behaviour occurs through observation, and often imitation, of other people's behaviour. Those people whose behaviour is observed and imitated can be described as role models. It could be argued, for example, that a child brought up in a family environment in which another family member suffers from and displays symptoms and behaviour consistent with anxiety, depression, or schizophrenia might in turn adopt these behaviours and patterns of thinking. Equally, children who are 'fussy eaters' may have observed and imitated the behaviour of parents who are dieting. Many people attribute the existence of a phobia (a severe fear of a specific object or situation) to observing and imitating a fear reaction by a parent confronted with the feared object or situation.

More recently, cognitive explanations of behaviour have been introduced to produce the cognitive–behavioural model, leading directly to cognitive–behaviour therapy as a therapeutic intervention. All of these interventions are further discussed in Chapter 7.

Cognitive model

Introduced in the 1950s, the cognitive model, which considers human thoughts and interpretations of thoughts to be the main determinants of behaviour, owes its origins in part to the rapid advancement in information technology in the latter half of the 20th century. For the first time, it became possible to design computer programs that could predict and mimic the ways in which humans might process information, for example during reasoning, problem solving, and decision making. Thus it became possible to begin to explain how these internal processes might operate in human beings.

Based on the belief that behaviour is determined by how individuals think about themselves and their world, mental health problems can be explained as being caused and maintained by errors or biases in thinking. These faulty and often irrational thoughts impair health function, so treatment aims to change faulty or dysfunctional thinking. Treatment approaches include the now well-known cognitive therapy developed by Aaron Beck (1989), sometimes combined with behavioural approaches to produce cognitive–behaviour therapy.

Humanistic model

The humanistic approach to explaining human behaviour and experience is sometimes described as the 'third force', as it was developed as an alternative to the view that human behaviour is determined either by unconscious forces and early experiences (as in the psychodynamic approach) or by external stimuli in the environment (as in the behavioural approach). The humanistic explanation, however, views humans as essentially positive beings, with the capacity for free will, for making choices, expressing values and determining their own purpose in life. Abraham Maslow's theory of human needs (Maslow 1954) illustrates this approach well. Maslow (1908–1970) was concerned with the meaning of existence, the identity of the individual, and the nature of the psychologically healthy person. In his theory, Maslow grouped human needs into categories, which were then prioritised into a hierarchy. This is commonly illustrated as a multi-layered triangle in which the categories of highest priority are the bottom-most layers.

Human beings are self-motivated to fulfil the lowest level of needs, at least in part, before needs higher up in the hierarchy may be addressed. Thus, physiological and safety needs must first be satisfied in order to ensure survival. Once these are satisfied, humans are motivated to satisfy their love and belonging needs, esteem needs, intellectual needs, aesthetic needs and the need for self-actualisation. Self-actualisation is the state whereby an individual has become the self that they want to be, but Maslow did allow for the fact that very few people actually achieve this desirable state, as we are almost always striving to achieve something more, or become something different or better.

The psychologist Carl Rogers (1902–1987) is often described as the father of humanistic psychology. Rogers (1961) supported Maslow's view that people have an 'actualising tendency' – a natural motivational force that is directed towards constructive growth. He adopted a non-mechanical, person-centred view of human nature, out of which developed the personal growth movement and the practices of person-centred counselling and encounter groups. This approach became popular in education, nursing, and other interpersonal professions during the 1960s and 1970s, and the counselling movement remains strong today.

Mental health problems, according to the humanistic viewpoint, might be explained as the result of people being thwarted in their efforts to grow and self-actualise. This may be due to environmental factors, or not being valued by other people, or being judged adversely by other people. The individual may then develop a negative self-concept, poor self-image, and low self-esteem, all of which are known to predispose to mental health problems.

Humanistic therapeutic interventions such as person-centred counselling are aimed at increasing the individual's capacity for personal responsibility and choice. The client, rather than the therapist, is seen as the expert, the therapist merely facilitates the individual's progress towards becoming their real self. Counselling is discussed further in Chapter 7.

Social models

As an alternative to medical and psychological explanations of mental health problems, there exists a range of explanations that consider problems to lie predominantly within the individual's social environment. These can be summarised as social models. As with behaviourism, social explanations consider that the causes of mental health problems lie firmly outside the person, in the individual's social world. In 1897 the sociologist Emile Durkheim showed that social factors were important in predicting suicide, in that the degree of cohesion in a group and the extent to which an individual felt part of that group affected the rate of suicide (Durkheim 1897/2002). When individuals' values became different from the society in which they lived, they would experience 'anomie', or a sense of alienation from society, which might lead them to choose suicide as a means of resolving this unpleasant experience.

More recently, Thomas Szasz (1960), a strong critic of the medicalisation of mental illness, suggested that mental illness did not really exist, rather that all individuals experience problems in living, through which they experience a continuous struggle for peace of mind. While the view that mental health problems do not exist may be thought extreme today, from the 1970s, there was certainly a great deal of support for the social model as a complete explanation of mental health problems, and a belief that environmental factors had more influence than any other factor as causes or precipitants of mental health problems. It is certainly true that problems reflect the society and culture in which we live. As an example, it is often thought that the high incidence of eating disorders (such as anorexia nervosa and bulimia nervosa) in industrialised Western societies may be due to the pressure put upon people, and particularly young women, to conform to a socially acceptable stereotype presented through the media – one that is often unnaturally thin. These eating disorders are rare in societies where food is in short supply and access to media images is restricted; for example, the fuller figure was the norm in Fiji until the advent of television in 1995, after which many adolescent girls began to show great interest in the slim Western figure, and a rise in eating disorders was noted (Becker et al 2002). However, there are likely to be many other factors, including genetic, personality, family, and social issues, involved in the development and maintenance of the complex problems involved in eating disorders, so we cannot solely blame Western society and its obsession with thinness for the incidence of these problems.

As a further example of the relationship between social factors and mental health problems, Brown & Harris (1978) claimed to have discovered a range of social causes of depression in their study of women living in a London borough. These included the lack of an intimate, confiding relationship; being a member of a lower social class; not having employment outside the home; and having a number of preschool children to care for at home. Other studies have drawn associations between mental health problems and unemployment, poverty, low social class, and low social status. These links may exist because people in these circumstances are likely to experience greater life stresses and have fewer support or coping strategies to help them resist or deal with stress factors.

In order to address problems produced by social and environmental factors, therapeutic interventions aim to bring about social and environmental changes. Examples of socially based therapeutic approaches include social psychiatry, the therapeutic community, and family therapy. In the latter half of the 20th century, some psychiatrists moved away from a focus on the individual to a focus on the relationship between individuals and their community. The therapeutic community movement, arising out of this new emphasis on social psychiatry, became popular in the 1960s and 1970s. Patients would be admitted, as in-patients or day patients, to an environment which was seen as a microcosm of society. Patients were jointly responsible for the day-to-day running of the community, along with staff members, and were active participants in their own and others' treatment (Bloom 1997). Hence, the community itself was the therapy, providing a secure, democratic, accepting, and empowering atmosphere in which individual members would experience social change and personal growth. Group therapies were used extensively. The therapeutic community movement continues today, and claims to be particularly successful in the treatment of people with personality disorders.

Family therapy is based on the idea that the family is a system, and that the behaviour of individuals and families is influenced and maintained by their interactions with other individuals and systems (Association for Family Therapy 2003). Hence, disturbances in a family will bring about disturbances in an individual within it, and vice versa. Thus, rather than focusing on the individual with a problem, the whole family is seen as 'the patient', and is assessed to try to discover and address the family dynamics that might be causing individual family members, or the family as a whole, to experience problems.

With the shift in focus in the care of people with mental health problems (with or without learning disabilities) from institutional to community care, the involvement of family members in care and treatment is now considered paramount to success. Family interventions are particularly successful in the prevention of relapse in people with schizophrenia. These and other socially based interventions are discussed further in Chapter 7.

Eclecticism and integrated approaches

There is a view that no one model or explanation of behaviour, and no one therapeutic approach, can be adequate in explaining and addressing the often complex problems experienced by individuals with mental health needs, and that a combination of approaches, from diverse sources, provides the most appropriate 'package' of understanding and responding to the problem. This view is known as eclecticism. The eclectic practitioner will draw upon whichever model or group of models of explanation and subsequent treatment seems most appropriate to address individual needs. For example, the now popular cognitive–behaviour therapy (see Ch. 7) is an integrated approach that combines two distinct models of explanation and treatment, often more successfully than either cognitive therapy or behaviour therapy alone. By the same token, acknowledging that there is likely to be a complex interplay of causative factors, people with schizophrenia are likely to be treated with a combination of medication, psychological, and family interventions. Therapeutic intervention strategies and packages for a wide range of mental health problems are discussed further in Chapter 7.

EXPLAINING MENTAL HEALTH PROBLEMS IN PEOPLE WITH LEARNING DISABILITIES

As we have seen in Chapter 1, people with learning disabilities experience the full range of mental health problems found in the general population, and many researchers have assumed that the fundamental causes of mental health problems in people with learning disabilities are similar to those in the general population. However, in the 1980s it was recognised that in some cases the sources of mental health problems in this client group might be different from those in the general population. Matson & Sevin (1994), for example, suggested four causal theories of mental health problems in people with learning disabilities: organic, behavioural, developmental, and sociocultural.

- The *organic* theory proposes that mental health problems in this client group have physiological origins, such as structural brain abnormalities or epilepsy; biochemical origins, such as those that predispose clients to schizophrenia or depression; or genetic causes, such as those produced through the established link between specific genetic disorders (e.g. Down's syndrome or fragile-X syndrome) and mental health problems.
- The *behavioural* model suggests that a person will develop certain behaviours as a result of complex relationships with their environment. For example, the client who is isolated and who has few self-help skills may become depressed.
- The *developmental* model proposes that cognitive ability develops universally within all humans, and that people with learning disabilities develop in the same way but at a much slower rate. A person's behaviour reflects underlying developmental structures. Therefore, behaviours that might be considered pathological for a person at a given chronological age may be considered normal for a person whose development is delayed, as in learning disabilities.

- The *sociocultural* model highlights the negative experiences that many people with learning disabilities have had during their life, which may culminate in them experiencing mental health problems.

As we saw in Chapter 1, history informs us of the segregation and negative value society has placed on these clients. Furthermore, we have seen the negative effects of institutional living, and also the stress experienced in moving out from institutions into community based facilities. Many people with learning disabilities experience discrimination in employment, housing, health services, relationships, and social activities.

We can see, therefore, that although people with learning disabilities are likely to share some aetiological factors with the general population, there are some specific genetic, developmental, and social features related to their learning disability that may help us to understand and explain the basis of mental health problems in this client group. However, whichever model or explanation we adopt, it is clearly necessary to identify and address the unique problems experienced by each individual in relation to their mental health needs.

Exercise
To return to the story of Jason with which this chapter opened, which, if any, of the models or explanations can help to explain his problems?

Jason's degree of learning disability is mild, but we do not know the reason for his disability. Some interesting research at the moment is exploring behavioural phenotypes. A behavioural phenotype is a group of specific behaviours associated with a genetic disorder – a group of behaviours resulting from an interaction between genes and the environment (see Ch. 3 for more detail on behavioural phenotypes). Hence it is possible that there is some genetic basis for Jason's difficulties, although it is likely that these would have manifested at a much earlier age, and produced more obvious symptoms and behaviours.

We do know that Jason's father had a 'nervous breakdown', so it is possible that Jason has inherited a set of genetic factors that might predispose him, too, to developing a mental health problem. In any case, at the age of 16, Jason is likely to be experiencing or has recently experienced the wide range of physical changes associated with puberty, which he may not fully understand or welcome. This may account for his current mood and behaviour. These factors would again support a biological or organic explanation for his difficulties.

However, we also know that Jason's father has left the family home, but we do not know how Jason feels about this. It may be that he is suffering from a delayed bereavement reaction, which would support a psychodynamic explanation for his current difficulties. It is widely acknowledged that bereavement amongst people with learning disabilities is a significant contributory factor in challenging behaviours and mental health problems (Read 2003). Jason may be worrying that he too will have a 'nervous breakdown' in the future; this might support the social learning explanation. We do not know, furthermore, how his father's absence has been explained to Jason. Perhaps he feels in some way to blame, that if he had been a better person or better behaved, his father would still be at home. These examples of faulty thinking would support the cognitive explanation. In addition, Jason has, up to now, attended a mainstream school, albeit with support, but at this crucial time in his life when exams are looming, he may be beginning to realise that his disability might prevent him from achieving particular goals in life, and he may be suffering from low self-esteem. This would support a humanistic explanation. In keeping with the psychodynamic model, as an adolescent, Jason may, in common with his non-learning disabled peers, be experiencing an 'identity crisis' (Erikson 1959), in which he is trying to establish himself as an individual independent of, and different from, his parents, and yet at the same time not wanting to leave the security and predictability of childhood. He may, in his own way, be rebelling against a lifestyle that he feels he has grown out of, or one that he has not chosen for himself.

At this time in his life, Jason is experiencing the effects of a range of external stress factors, such as losing his job and income, and having to make important decisions about his future. This would support a social explanation for his difficulties.

So, even though Jason has a mild learning disability, it is likely that the cause of his mental health problems, if indeed he has any, is similar to anyone else in the population as a whole. However, as Matson & Sevin (1994) showed, people with learning disabilities are often particularly predisposed to experience mental health problems due to a range of particular vulnerability factors.

Exercise

Can you identify any factors in Jason's life that may have made him particularly vulnerable to developing a mental health problem?

Vulnerability factors

People with learning disabilities can experience a range of vulnerability factors that make them particularly susceptible to developing mental health problems. Prenatal brain damage, birth injury, intellectual disability, and low intelligence are all, in themselves, risk factors for the development of mental health problems. Other factors may be features of the learning disability itself; for example, if individuals have limited or non-existent speech, then it will be difficult for them to communicate their distress to others in a readily accessible way. They are likely, then, literally to suffer in silence, if carers are not adept at picking up other signs and manifestations of distress, and interpreting them accurately.

Furthermore, people with learning disabilities have often experienced a range of adverse life events that predispose them to mental health problems. These might include long-term institutionalisation, repeated losses through home moves, or frequent change of carers, or family difficulties and rejection. They may have been bereaved, and yet not have been helped to understand or express their feelings about their loss. They may experience low self-esteem through failure to achieve things seen as desirable in society, such as a job or a meaningful relationship. If they have lived in an over-protective environment they may not have developed their own coping strategies to draw upon in the face of stress, and they may have experienced labelling, stigmatisation, exploitation or abuse to a greater extent than people in the general population. It is known that people with learning disabilities experience extensive degrees of many forms of abuse including physical, emotional, and financial, and are at a higher risk of experiencing sexual abuse than the general population (Cambridge 1998). This may result in low self-esteem, low self-confidence, depression, anxiety, aggression, self-harm, and difficulties in forming trusting relationships (Sant Angelo 2000). They may lack consistent sources of social support, which is known to be a strongly protective factor in preventing or reducing the effects of depression and other mental health problems. They may have poor social networks generally. Equally, they are likely to have a dependent role in relationships with other people and lack assertiveness in interactions. Finally, they may have lived in less than ideal environments, with little control over choice of fellow residents, physical surroundings, activities, and structure of the day, and may have experienced lack of privacy in carrying out their daily activities.

All of these factors (loss, change, low self-esteem, abuse, exploitation, lack of social support, lack of control, poor coping skills, and adverse environments) are known to predispose to mental ill health in the general population. It is clear, then, that people with learning disabilities are at least as likely, if not more likely, to experience mental ill health than members of the general population. However, as we saw in Chapter 1, and will explore further in Chapter 3, the emotional needs of people with learning disabilities have long gone unrecognised.

In Jason's case, apart from experiencing a major loss in his life, there do not appear to be too many other vulnerability factors that might have contributed to or exacerbated his problems, and a word of caution is needed here. It must not be assumed that all people with learning disabilities are vulnerable in this way. Northway (2002) describes the concept 'vulnerable' as meaning something that can be wounded or harmed, if it is exposed to damage without adequate protection. Although no-one lives a life that is free from risk, there is always the possibility that harm can be avoided. Thus, rather than making the assumption that people with learning disabilities will inevitably be vulnerable to mental health problems, we should aim to prevent and reduce vulnerability rather than dealing with its effects.

Exercise

Can you think of any ways in which Jason is protected from being vulnerable to mental health problems?

The fact that Jason has a close circle of friends and appears to have support from his mother could be protective factors. He may also have a supportive relationship with his learning support teacher at school. Furthermore, he has, until recently, made a contribution to society (or at least to the family's income) through his Saturday job, and been rewarded for his efforts. It would appear, from his participation in sporting activities, that he is physically fit and healthy. Social support, meaningful relationships, physical well-being, and increased self-esteem are all known to protect people from (or at least minimise the effects of) stress, loss, and change to some degree, so in this respect Jason's future, whatever his mental health status turns out to be, is not as bleak as it might be for others.

CONCLUSION

In this chapter we have explored a range of explanations for the occurrence of mental health problems in the general population and considered the appropriateness of these explanations in relation to people with learning disabilities. In conclusion, while people with learning disabilities may be exposed to many of the same risk factors for mental health problems as people in the general population, they may have additional physical, psychological, and social risk factors that increase their vulnerability. To compound the issue, they may also lack some of the compensating factors which many people draw upon to help deal with their problems. Strategies aimed at preventing and reducing vulnerability to mental health problems in people with learning disabilities, and thereby promoting their mental health, are discussed further in Chapter 8.

In Chapter 3, we explore some of the difficulties in identifying and accurately assessing mental health problems when they are experienced by people with learning disabilities.

REFERENCES

American Psychiatric Association 1994 Diagnostic and statistical manual of mental disorders DSM-IV, 4th edn. American Psychiatric Association, Washington

American Psychiatric Association 2000 Diagnostic and statistical manual of mental disorders DSM-IV-TR (Text Revision). American Psychiatric Association, Washington

Association for Family Therapy and Systemic Practice in the UK 2003 What is family therapy? Online. Available: http://www.aft.org.uk

Beck A T 1989 Cognitive therapy and the emotional disorders. Penguin, Harmondsworth

Becker A, Burwell R, Gilman S 2002 Eating behaviour and attitudes following prolonged exposure to television among ethnic Fijian adolescent girls. British Journal of Psychiatry 180: 509–514

Bloom S L 1997 The therapeutic community. Online. Available: http://www.sanctuaryweb.com/main/therapeutic_community

Brown G W, Harris T 1978 The social origins of depression. Tavistock, London

Cambridge P 1998 The physical abuse of people with learning disabilities and challenging behaviours: lessons for commissioners and providers. Tizard Learning Disability Review 3(1): 18–26

Durkheim E 2002 Suicide: a study in sociology. Routledge, London (Original work published 1897)

Erikson E 1959 Identity and the life cycle. Norton, New York

Maslow A H 1954 Motivation and personality. Harper and Row, New York

Matson J L, Sevin J A 1994 Theories of dual diagnosis in mental retardation. Journal of Consulting and Clinical Psychology 62(1): 6–16

Northway R 2002 The nature of vulnerability. Learning Disability Practice 5(6): 26

Read S 2003 Bereavement and loss. In: Marwick A, Parrish A (eds) Learning disabilities. Themes and perspectives. Butterworth Heinemann, Edinburgh, p 81–109

Rogers C 1961 On becoming a person: a therapist's view of psychotherapy. Houghton Mifflin, Boston

Sant Angelo D 2000 Learning disability community nursing: addressing emotional and sexual health needs. In: Astor R, Jefferys K (eds) Positive initiatives for people with learning difficulties. Macmillan, Basingstoke, p 52–68

Szasz T S 1960 The myth of mental illness. American Psychologist 15: 113–118

World Health Organization 1992 ICD-10: The international statistical classification of diseases and related health problems, 10th revision. WHO, Geneva

FURTHER READING

Joseph S 2001 Psychopathology and therapeutic approaches. An introduction. Palgrave, Basingstoke

3

Assessing the mental health needs of people with learning disabilities

INTRODUCTION

Thus far we have examined some of the theories and issues surrounding the concept of mental health in people with learning disabilities, and have traced the historical development of relevant ideas, attitudes, and explanatory theories in relation to people with learning disabilities and those with mental health problems. We have touched upon some of the difficulties in explaining, identifying, and addressing mental health problems in people with learning disabilities, and in this chapter we explore those difficulties in greater depth. In particular, we discuss the concept of diagnostic overshadowing, and the difficulties of distinguishing between challenging behaviour and mental ill health, both of which can present barriers to effective assessment. We also explore the effects of inadequate staff knowledge and training, assessment tools, and service provision on assessment of mental health needs. Particular attention will be paid to the challenges of assessment when clients have severe or profound learning disabilities, and to focus our attention on some of these issues we begin by presenting the case study of Jenny.

Case study: Jenny

Jenny, aged 34, lives with her mother, older sister and her sister's husband and their two young children in a four-bedroomed house. Her mother has always attended to all her daily and personal needs. At school Jenny was labelled as having severe learning disabilities. As a child she would urinate over her sister's belongings, be cruel to any pets that were in the home, and constantly pick at her skin until it bled. To occupy Jenny, her mother would let her watch the television and videos in her room. As a young adult her behaviour is now exaggerated. She is very destructive to property, self-mutilates, and will attempt to pinch and bite people around her. These exaggerated problems have increased over the last few years such that the family can no longer cope with her behaviours, and Jenny has been admitted for a 12-week

---

period of assessment to a unit that specialises in helping people who display challenging behaviour. The staff have observed that she constantly bites and tears at her fingernails, and when prevented from doing this she becomes very aggressive to people around her. Her communication skills are limited and she is often heard screaming. She does, however, use very basic sign language. Staff have recently noticed that she has become selective in what she eats. They have carried out observations and are about to complete a functional analysis with the aim of implementing a behaviourally based care programme.

Exercise

- What do you think might be happening to Jenny?
- What should the care team be doing prior to implementing a programme of care?
- How might the fact that Jenny has severe learning disabilities affect the assessment process?

ASSESSMENT AND DIAGNOSIS

The content of this chapter should help us to begin to answer the above questions. In Jenny's case, a diagnosis would be very useful to help give focus to future care planning and interventions. But what happens if the diagnosis is wrong? Will treatment regimes and care delivery then be ineffective? Would Jenny then suffer unnecessarily? Are there needs in her life that are unmet? For people with learning disabilities, there are particular challenges in arriving at an accurate identification of mental health needs. As shown in Chapter 1, people with learning disabilities are at an increased risk of experiencing emotional problems compared with the general population. Furthermore, Moss (1995) demonstrated that this client group is at an even higher risk for psychosis, autism, and challenging behaviour. However, difficulties are less likely to be accurately identified in people with learning disabilities than in the general population. White et al (1995) suggest that people with learning disabilities can expect a 19% drop in diagnostic accuracy and treatment for mental health problems, in contrast to people with the same mental health problems but without learning disabilities.

People with learning disabilities like Jenny are at a disadvantage in relation to an accurate mental health diagnosis as they already have a multitude of complexities and problems in their life, together with needs that are not ordinarily associated with people of the same age. For the person with mild learning disabilities there may be problems related to social inclusion, education, employment, and relationships. Whilst the person with severe learning disabilities may have problems with independent functioning skills, or lack of communication skills, these problems are compounded when it is identified that they also have a mental health problem. There are now at least two diagnosable conditions.

Most clinicians, carers and families welcome a diagnosis; it sets the scene for the future. If the carer knows what the problems are, then a particular care regime can be implemented. Assessment and history taking are key to any diagnostic and treatment plan. A detailed history will set a client's needs into a context within which the client and the care providers can plan appropriate care (Levitas & Silka 2001). Usually diagnosis begins with the client's description of their emotional experiences. However, in people who have learning disabilities it is not always possible to gain at first hand a reliable history or description, particularly if such individuals lack the ability to communicate verbally, or lack the cognitive ability to describe emotions. This is a major barrier to assessment and diagnosis and could lead to the assumption on the part of the assessor that clients cannot have a mental health problem. Hence the clinician must turn to families and carers for an account of clients' emotional state. It is here that the key skill of listening is paramount. The assessor can then try to place the details of the account into context with other psychopathology that presents in recognised mental health problems, and so determine which symptoms are present and which are not.

A note of caution must be made here. Bramston & Fogarty (2000) suggest that there are three common methodologies used for the assessment of mental health problems in people with learning disabilities:

- ratings by a 'significant other' such as a carer, family member, or professional carer
- a clinical interview, normally completed by a professional carer
- self-reporting by the client.

Assessors need to be aware that the three methodologies sometimes provide conflicting data, and therefore must utilise a range of methods to collect sufficient information upon which an accurate assessment can be confidently made.

The recognition of mental health problems in people with learning disabilities

The recognition of mental health problems in people with learning disabilities is often a difficult process. Twenty years ago it was recognised that mental health problems were more likely to go unnoticed in people with learning disabilities than in the general population (Marston et al 1997). Reiss et al (1982) and Sovner (1986) provide some explanations, as outlined below, but there are many potential barriers to the effective assessment and diagnosis of mental health problems in people with learning disabilities. These include diagnostic overshadowing; clients' communication and linguistic abilities; lack of appropriate assessment tools; inadequate service provision; poor staff knowledge; difficulties in distinguishing between challenging behaviour and mental health problems; and the relationship between behavioural phenotypes and challenging behaviours. All of these potential barriers to assessment are discussed below.

Diagnostic overshadowing and related diagnostic difficulties

In returning to Jenny, you may have identified that some of the symptoms that she exhibits could be attributed either to a mental health problem or to her learning disabilities. In Chapter 1 we introduced the concept of *diagnostic overshadowing*, that is, when behaviours presented by a client which might be indicative of mental health problems are attributed instead to the symptoms of the person's learning disabilities (Reiss et al 1982), or when the salience of the client's cognitive deficits impacts negatively on the clinician's judgement of the client's mental health state (Jopp & Keys 2001). Hence the diagnosis of learning disabilities and its problems takes priority over emotional problems. The concept is not new; in fact diagnostic overshadowing was first used to explain the underdiagnosis of mental health problems such as schizophrenia, but the literature on diagnostic overshadowing suggests that it is a common phenomenon, and hence people's needs may still be overlooked because of its influence.

Sovner (1986) provides further explanation for the lack of recognition of mental health problems in people with learning disabilities, by identifying four areas that may lead to confusion. The first area is the relatively low level of skills and functioning of many people with learning disabilities, leading to reduced ability to express or communicate internal feelings. This is described as *intellectual distortion*, and it can lead to a decrease in the effectiveness of the diagnostic tools that utilise direct communication between the client and the clinician, who will have difficulty in gaining objective evidence of symptoms. Reliance on subjective observations made by the family and other carers, although valuable, can lead to a dilution of objective information. In Jenny's case, she can communicate using basic sign language, but this may not help her to convey her emotional state.

The second area of difficulty is *psychological masking*. This is where the client's life experience may be limited compared to that of the general population, and thus the mental health symptoms may not appear to be as significant as they might in a person without learning disabilities. For example, clients who have lived in an institutional setting, or who have lived with over-protective parents, may have had their everyday needs such as clothing, activities, health care, and accommodation provided for them, and will thus have a limited experience of life. This is certainly true of Jenny's situation. Compare this with the life of non-learning disabled people of the same age who have been brought up in a more independent way, and who have a wealth of experiences to call upon, especially when attempting to communicate their emotions. However, the clinician must also take into account that many people with learning disabilities are able to mimic the life experiences and behaviours of their carers, and may therefore appear to have more experience of life than they actually have.

The third area is known as *cognitive disintegration*, and is where, for example, anxiety becomes overwhelming and acts to disorganise thought processes such that it overpowers how the client thinks, feels and acts.

The final area of difficulty is *baseline exaggeration*, which has similar effects to diagnostic overshadowing. This describes the increase in cognitive deficits and negative behaviour that may be a result of the co-morbid state of learning disabilities and mental health problems. Instead of the increase in cognitive deficits and negative behaviours being attributed to the new mental health state they are attributed instead to the original problem behaviours that the client may have been expressing prior to any change in their mental health status. It could be, for example, that carers will relate Jenny's new behaviours of biting and tearing at her fingernails to previous behaviours such as skin picking, and not consider that Jenny may be trying to communicate some of her emotional needs in this new way.

Communication and linguistic abilities

Assuming that mental health problems are suspected in a person with learning disabilities, there are other barriers that can inhibit an objective diagnosis. The process of assessment itself can often be difficult, particularly if clients have communication or linguistic difficulties. It is recognised that people with mild to moderate learning disabilities can benefit from mainstream approaches to their mental health problems. Assessment tools designed for the general population can be used to aid arrival at an accurate diagnosis and the instigation of conventional treatment regimes. People with mild to moderate learning disabilities generally have better linguistic and communication skills and may be very well able to articulate their thoughts and ideas. However, clients with severe learning disabilities may have few or absent linguistic skills and poor abstract cognitive abilities, and so face many barriers in the effective assessment of mental health problems. Assessment and diagnosis rely heavily on the client's communication ability. If the client cannot communicate emotions, then there is a strong chance that the appropriate care and intervention will not be received. Often the assessment is completed by a third party who knows the client, perhaps a care worker or family member, and they may omit important issues that they are not aware of or misinterpret.

Even when clients' mental health needs have been recognised, lack of communication skills can still be a barrier to effective assessment. They may have a limited vocabulary or communicate only using sign language or pictorial methods of communication. A further barrier is the potential for misunderstanding of the meaning of words. For example, Eric, who had been admitted to a respite service, told his carers that he was depressed. After spending a period of time with Eric, the key worker felt that the client did not have the signs or symptoms of depression, and when the client was asked what he meant by depression he said that the care staff were getting at him to do jobs around the home. The client's meaning of depression was completely different from that of the professional carers. After further discussions with Eric it was discovered that one of his relatives had been diagnosed with depression and that he was merely repeating what he had overheard in conversations.

In another case, Gloria informed the care staff that she was hearing voices telling her what to do. It was eventually discovered that she was actually 'thinking aloud', but had been influenced by hearing a psychiatrist explain to an inexperienced carer what hallucinations were, and believed that her normal cognitive experiences were in some way problematic.

These two examples demonstrate that clients sometimes convey a deeper or different understanding of their emotional state than they may actually experience.

Assessment tools

If interventions are to be successful, then a comprehensive assessment must be carried out, and one of the hallmarks of good practice is to base care upon reliable and valid data. The process of obtaining such data can be assisted by the use of appropriate assessment tools, and while the use of tools can be time consuming, the results can prove very valuable to the client. There is a range of tools available for the assessment of mental health problems in people with learning disabilities. Some clinicians and researchers have adopted tools used in the general population and applied them in learning disabilities settings, such as the KGV Manchester Scale (Krawiecka et al 1977). Others have adapted tools; for example, Lindsay & Michie (1988) have adapted the Zung Self-rating Anxiety Scale (Zung 1971) for use with people with learning disabilities. Other tools have been developed specifically for people with learning disabilities, such as the DASH-II (Matson 1995), PAS-ADD (Moss et al 1996), ADD (Matson & Bamburg 1998), CANDID (Xenitidis et al 2000), and the LDCNS (Raghavan et al 2001). These tools are discussed in detail in Chapter 6, but one problem related to the use of such tools could be lack of training and experience of those attempting to use them.

A further difficulty is that we still have some way to go until all of these tools can be verified as accurate, valid, and reliable, especially for people with severe and profound learning disabilities (Ross & Oliver 2003). Hamer (1998) proposes a framework that, when the carer is ready to assess a client, could help in the assessment process. JOMAAC – an acronym for judgement, orientation, memory, affect, attitude, and cognition – is a quick reference guide designed in response to the needs of the client.

Service provision

Service provision can sometimes create a barrier to effective assessment. The issue of who provides services for people with learning disabilities who have mental health needs is a contentious one. Many people would agree that the mental health needs of people with learning disables are too complex for any one service to respond to effectively, and that there should be specialist services that provide highly developed skills and expertise (Barlow 1999, Oliver et al 2003), to include expertise in assessment. The Mansell Report (Department of Health 1993) recommended that such services should be provided locally and be tailor-made for individual needs. However, it is more usual for authorities to provide discrete mental health and learning disabilities services, and there are few examples where both services complement one another. Often clients with learning disabilities are not accepted into general mental health services, as these services do not have the appropriate resources to cater for people with an IQ below 70. More recently partnership boards have attempted to create multi-agency and complementary services, which should ensure a more appropriate assessment process. These issues are discussed further in Chapter 9.

Staff knowledge and training

The most usual way in which physical and mental health problems are detected in the general population is through a visit to a family doctor or general practitioner (GP) (Bramston & Fogarty 2000). While this may be adequate for the non-learning disabled population, many GPs in the UK acknowledge that the physical health care needs of people with learning disabilities are less well met than those of the general population, and that they would welcome training in this field (Singh 1997). This is likely also to be true for GPs' knowledge of the mental health needs of people with learning disabilities, and true also for other health and social care practitioners. However, contrary to this, Day (1999) suggests that both GPs and psychiatrists are well informed about learning disabilities in that their training has several components devoted to such areas. Furthermore, other professions such as social work and psychology have input into their training relating to learning disabilities, supported by work placements in relevant services.

However, whether or not such professionals have the appropriate knowledge in relation to the health needs of people with learning disabilities, it is clear that staff working directly with people with learning disabilities sometimes lack knowledge in relation to the mental health needs of their clients, which creates potential for inadequate assessment and identification of problem areas. In recent studies by Bates et al (2004) and Quigley et al (2001) it was demonstrated that many staff caring for people with learning disabilities had not received any training in mental health, even though training was felt to be an important factor in relation to assessing and responding to mental health issues.

Within the nursing profession in the UK, there has been specialist training leading to a qualification in learning disabilities nursing for over 50 years, which has, over this period, responded to philosophical, political and care changes, moving from a medical base to a social care base. However, although current learning disabilities nurse education programmes do include some attention to mental health issues, it is unlikely that much time is available to devote to the subject within the skills-based curricula advocated by professional bodies (Department of Health 1999, UKCC 1999). A number of nurses in the learning disabilities field have also gained mental health nursing qualifications, although anecdotal evidence suggests that they find difficulty in bridging the gap between the two fields, both in relation to service provision and treatment regimes. Those nurses in learning disabilities settings who have gained relevant skills and knowledge are likely to have done so by attendance at short courses or 'in-house' study days, but there is no systematic national programme to ensure that such training occurs, nor to govern the content of such programmes. Carers working in social care settings are even less likely to have received any mental health training than those working in health care settings (Bates et al 2004), and carers who are not professionally qualified (significant numbers of whom care for people with learning disabilities) are even less likely to receive training and hence lack knowledge, understanding and skills to recognise and respond to mental health needs in the client group than their professionally qualified colleagues (Bates et al 2004, Gibbs & Priest 1999).

A further difficulty is that if symptoms of mental health problems are not disruptive to services, then there is less likelihood that they will be regarded as problems by carers, and therefore not investigated as potential mental health problems (Marston et al 1997). Taggart & McConkey (2001), too, showed that staff were less consistent in observing less serious behaviours. Their study aimed to discover whether 'front-line' care staff differed in their assessments of the same clients. Though only a small sample was used, the results indicated that care staff were consistent in observing severe problems but not in less serious problems. Taggart & McConkey (2001) also suggested that there is a lack of inter-rater and inter-observer reliability even when standardised assessment tools are used, and staff can still make subjective judgements regarding clients' behaviour, which may confound the results of such tools. The lack of recognition of signs and symptoms of mental health problems in clients by care staff further compounds the clients' situation, if this means that they are not referred to the relevant specialist.

Distinguishing between challenging behaviour and mental health problems

Chapter 1 identified some problems in ascertaining accurate prevalence rates for mental health problems in people with learning disabilities. A key issue is whether or not challenging behaviours are viewed as a form of mental health problem. Moss et al (2000) attempted to determine what proportion of people with learning disabilities actually had mental health problems. Their results indicate that there is a significant association between the two and that in certain conditions people with learning disabilities and challenging behaviours also have unrecognised mental health problems. This association is significant in that the way behaviour is viewed will determine prevalence rates for mental health problems, assessment strategies, treatments and interventions, and service provision.

Challenging behaviour can be difficult to define. It could be argued that the term itself is a negative label and thus portrays a negative image of people who challenge services due to their unique needs. The concept of challenging behaviour can be viewed as a social construct which is defined by the impact the construct has on the clients and the service. Hence definitions of challenging behaviour vary widely, but may be best described as the ways in which people try to gain control over difficult situations (Department of Health 2001). In attempting to define severely challenging behaviour, Emerson (1995) suggests that it is either behaviour of such intensity, frequency or duration that the physical safety of the client or others is placed in serious jeopardy, or behaviour which is likely to seriously limit or deny clients access to the use of ordinary community facilities. Challenging behaviours vary widely and can include violence and aggression, antisocial behaviour, withdrawal, stereotyped and odd mannerisms, self-abusive behaviour, and hyperactivity.

Challenging behaviour has a major consequence for clients. They may be a danger to themselves and/or others, and hence their lifestyle in relation to where they live, how they live, and with whom they live is compromised. The behaviour also has adverse effects on their social activity and the kinds of occupation in which they may participate. It also has consequences for service providers. Modern service providers work within the framework of rights, independence, choice and inclusion. The Mansell Committee (Department of Health 1993) stressed that services for people with challenging behaviours should be commissioned on an individual basis and should seek to promote inclusive lifestyles. Catering for the needs of people who present significant challenges is one of the major issues facing learning disabilities service providers (Department of Health 2001).

As we have indicated, some challenging behaviour may be associated with mental health disorder, which has an impact not just in ascertaining prevalence rates but also on the accurate assessment of clients' mental health needs. Emerson et al (1999) identify possible ways in which mental health problems can be associated with challenging behaviours. For example, challenging behaviour may be viewed as an atypical presentation of a mental health disorder. Emerson et al (1999) cite as an example the person with severe learning disabilities who self-injures. Self-injurious behaviour and obsessive–compulsive behaviours share some similarities in that both can involve repetitive and ritualistic behaviour; hence the skill of the assessor is to have an understanding of such atypical presentations and to interpret behaviour accurately. Secondly, challenging behaviour may be a secondary feature of a mental health problem. For example, a client with severe learning disabilities who is suffering from depression may become agitated or aggressive as a means of expressing emotional distress. Finally, mental health problems may be functional in that a client may develop them, perhaps unconsciously, in order to adapt to a particular situation.

An understanding of the relationship between challenging behaviour and mental health problems can be useful in developing underpinning theory and positive care regimes. Above all, carers must keep an open mind when working with people whose behaviour is challenging in some way, and try to explore all possible explanations for that behaviour in the light of existing and developing knowledge.

Behavioural phenotypes and challenging behaviours

As an example of developing knowledge, there has, in recent years, been a growing recognition that some challenging behaviours can be associated with genetic conditions. For example, people with Lesch–Nyhan syndrome (see Ch. 5), although appearing to be normal at birth, often develop self-injurious behaviour, particularly by gnawing their knuckles and biting their lips. Recent advances in molecular genetics have made it possible to identify specific genetic loci for conditions associated with learning disabilities, and it is now possible to identify a constellation of behaviours that are associated with particular genetic conditions. These associations are referred to as *behavioural phenotypes*. Down was the first to identify such phenotypes; he described people with Down's syndrome as having strong powers of imitation, a lively character, and a good sense of humour. Though this has been criticised as being too simplistic and generalised, there is some evidence that many people with Down's syndrome are in fact particularly sociable (Dykens et al 1994).

Holland (1999) argues that recognising the links between specific causes of learning disabilities and behavioural phenotypes may guide clinical intervention in some cases. There is still confusion, however, about behavioural phenotypes, as some behaviour occurs in several genetic loci. Furthermore, the research methods used to identify them are sometimes flawed or based purely on individual case studies. Hence if we are unaware of the associations, or do not have adequate evidence, the process of assessment and adapting to clients' specific needs may be impeded.

CASE STUDY REFLECTIONS

In bringing together the issues discussed in this chapter we can now return to Jenny and see that she is presenting very complex needs that will require an equally complex approach to assessment and intervention. The questions presented are difficult to answer. We cannot simply say that Jenny has a mental health problem. She could be exhibiting behavioural problems that are associated with her particular learning disability, or which she has learned from imitating other people. The services in which she has been assessed may not be adequately trained to understand the concept of mental health in people with learning disabilities, and may not have appropriate tools and resources to assist in the assessment process. Diagnostic overshadowing may be a barrier to her care.

Jenny will need a comprehensive assessment within the context of the family environment to which she will return; however, as she has complex needs including severe disability, poor communication skills and challenging behaviour, the assessment process will be difficult. Individualised non-verbal communication aids such as picture boards, books, and computer programs could be used to help her to express her feelings. Jenny's carers in the assessment unit have, commendably, commenced the process of identifying her particular problems, and what might be causing and maintaining them, by means of functional analysis; however it is likely that she will also benefit from the use of assessment tools designed to identify underlying mental health problems that can be carried out by her carers, such as the PAS-ADD tools or tools designed for people with severe levels of disability such as the DASH-II (see Ch. 6), which might identify the broad areas in which she has problems, and highlight the need for referral to an appropriate mental health professional.

CONCLUSION

Assessing the mental health needs of people with learning disabilities is fraught with complications. There are many skilled professionals that can carry out comprehensive mental health assessments in the general population; however there are only a limited number of experts in the field of learning disabilities. We have shown throughout this chapter that there are many barriers facing both clients and their carers in relation to the assessment of mental health needs. Carers need to be aware of these potential barriers, and especially those that impact on the assessment of clients with severe learning disabilities. In particular, they need to understand the concepts of diagnostic overshadowing and the difficulty in distinguishing between mental health and behaviour problems. Communication methods need to be developed, and the use of non-verbal communication systems may need to be introduced into the assessment of mental health needs. For example, expression through picture boards, books, and drama may be used to overcome some of the barriers. Education for carers is imperative if clients are to benefit from mental health assessment. The development of partnerships needs to be encouraged so that experts and family members can work together in order to produce objective, meaningful assessments that will lead to a clear diagnosis and a comprehensive package of care.

REFERENCES

Barlow C 1999 Issues in the management of clients with the dual diagnosis of learning disabilities and mental illness. Journal of Learning Disabilities for Nursing, Health and Social Care 3(3): 159–162

Bates P, Priest H, Gibbs M 2004 Education and training needs of learning disability staff in relation to mental health issues. Nurse Education in Practice (in press)

Bramston P, Fogarty G 2000 The assessment of emotional distress experienced by people with intellectual disability: a study of different methodologies. Research in Developmental Disabilities 21: 487–500

Day K 1999 Service provision and staff training. An overview. In: Došen A, Day K (eds) Treating mental illness and behavior disorders in children and adults with mental retardation. American Psychiatric Press, Washington, p 469–492

Department of Health 1993 Challenging behaviours and/or mental health needs of people with learning disabilities (Mansell report). HMSO, London

Department of Health 1999 Making a difference. Strengthening the nursing, midwifery and health visitor contribution to health and healthcare. Department of Health, London

Department of Health 2001 Valuing people: a new strategy for learning disabilities for the 21st century. Department of Health, London

Dykens E, Hodapp R, Evans E 1994 Profiles and development of adaptive behaviour in children with Down syndrome. American Journal on Mental Retardation 89: 580–587

Emerson E 1995 Challenging behaviour: analysis and interventions in people with learning difficulties. Cambridge University Press, Cambridge

Emerson E, Moss S, Kiernan C 1999 The relationship between challenging behaviour and psychiatric disorders in people with severe developmental disabilities. In: Bouras N (ed) Psychiatric and behavioural disorders in developmental disabilities and mental retardation. Cambridge University Press, Cambridge, p 38–48

Gibbs M, Priest H M 1999 Designing and implementing a dual diagnosis module: a review of the literature and some preliminary findings. Nurse Education Today 19: 357–363

Hamer B A 1998 Assessing mental health status in persons with mental retardation. Journal of Psychosocial Nursing 36(5): 27–31

Holland A 1999 Syndromes, phenotypes and genotypes: finding the links. The Psychologist 12(5): 242–245

Jopp D, Keys C B 2001 Diagnostic overshadowing reviewed and reconsidered. American Journal on Mental Retardation 106(5): 416–433

Krawiecka M, Goldberg D, Vaughan M 1977 A standardised psychiatric assessment scale for rating chronic psychotic patients. Acta Psychiatrica Scandinavica 55: 299–308

Levitas A S, Silka Van R 2001 Mental health clinical assessment of persons with mental retardation and developmental disabilities: history. Mental Health Aspects of Developmental Disabilities 4(1): 31–42

Lindsay W R, Michie A M 1988 Adaptation of the Zung self-rating anxiety scale for people with a mental handicap. Journal of Mental Deficiency Research 32: 485–490

Marston G M, Perry D W, Roy A 1997 Manifestations of depression in people with intellectual disability. Journal of Intellectual Disability Research 41(6): 476–480

Matson J L 1995 The diagnostic assessment for the severely handicapped II. Scientific Publishers, Baton Rouge

Matson J L, Bamburg J W 1998 Reliability of the assessment of dual diagnosis (ADD). Research in Developmental Disabilities 19(1): 89–95

Moss S 1995 Methodological issues in the diagnosis of psychiatric disorders in adults with learning disabilities. Thornfield Journal (University of Dublin) 18: 9–18

Moss S, Goldberg D, Patel P et al 1996 The psychiatric assessment schedule for adults with a developmental disability: PAS-ADD. Hester Adrian Research Centre, Manchester

Moss S, Emerson E, Kiernan C et al 2000 Psychiatric symptoms in adults with learning disabilities and challenging behaviour. British Journal of Psychiatry 177: 453–456

Oliver P, Piachaud J, Regan A et al 2003 Difficulties developing evidence-based approaches in learning disabilities. Evidence-Based Mental Health 6: 37–39

Quigley A, Murray G C, McKenzie K et al 2001 Staff knowledge about symptoms of mental health problems in people with learning disabilities. Journal of Learning Disabilities 5(3): 235–244

Raghavan R, Marshall M, Lockwood A et al 2001 The learning disabilities version of the cardinal needs schedule (LDCNS) (unpublished; available from r.raghavan@bradford.ac.uk)

Reiss S, Levitan G W, Szyszko J 1982 Emotional disturbance and mental retardation: diagnostic overshadowing. American Journal of Mental Deficiency 86: 567–574

Ross E, Oliver C 2003 The assessment of mood in adults who have severe or profound mental retardation. Clinical Psychology Review 23: 234–245

Singh P 1997 Preparation for change. Mencap, London

Sovner R 1986 Limiting factors in the use of DSM-III criteria with mentally ill/mentally retarded persons. Psychopharmacology Bulletin 24(4): 1055–1059

Taggart L, McConkey R 2001 The assessment of challenging behaviours in people with learning disabilities. Mental Health Care 4(7): 228–232

UKCC 1999 Fitness for practice. The UKCC commission for nursing and midwifery education. The United Kingdom Central Council for Nursing, Midwifery and Health Visiting, London

White M J, Nichols C N, Cook R S et al 1995 Diagnostic overshadowing and mental retardation: a meta-analysis. American Journal on Mental Retardation 100(3): 293–298

Xenitidis K, Thornicroft G, Leese M et al 2000 Reliability and validity of the CANDID – a needs assessment instrument for adults with learning disabilities and mental health problems. British Journal of Psychiatry 176: 473–478

Zung W K 1971 A rating instrument for anxiety disorders. Psychosomatics 12: 371–379

4

Common mental health problems experienced by people with learning disabilities

INTRODUCTION

As has been shown in previous chapters, people with learning disabilities experience the full range of mental health problems found in the population as a whole. Furthermore, they experience a diverse range of life problems and concerns (Prout & Stromer 1998). Amongst the aims put forward in *The Health of the Nation: A Strategy for People with Learning Disabilities* (Department of Health 1995) was a reduction in ill health and death caused by mental illness. The first step towards achieving this aim is for carers to have an understanding of the range of mental health problems commonly experienced in the general population; how these problems are manifested; and to what extent these manifestations are the same as or different in people with learning disabilities. In this way, carers may be better equipped to recognise and respond to actual or potential mental health problems in their clients.

This chapter, therefore, describes commonly occurring mental health problems, including mood disorders, anxiety disorders, and schizophrenia. Additionally, a section focuses on the mental health needs of older people, with specific reference to the relationship between Alzheimer's disease and Down's syndrome. Prevalence and manifestations of these problems in people with learning disabilities will be discussed, with particular attention to manifestations that are different from those in the general population. Implications from clients' and carers' perspectives will be discussed.

CLASSIFYING MENTAL HEALTH PROBLEMS

As noted in Chapter 1, the American Psychiatric Association (1994, p xxi) provides us with a clear definition of mental disorder:

…a clinically significant behavioral or psychological syndrome or pattern that occurs in an individual and that is associated with present distress or disability or with a significantly increased risk of suffering, death, pain, disability, or an important loss of freedom.

In order to help them to understand, label and treat these 'significant behavioural or psychological syndromes or patterns' that are presented in clinics and hospitals, psychiatrists typically draw upon one of two key diagnostic tools: ICD-10 (World Health Organization 1992) or DSM-IV (American Psychiatric Association 1994, 2000). These diagnostic tools, which are described in greater depth in Chapter 6, are complex, and require many years of medical training and experience before they can be used. Therefore, a simpler classification system may be more useful to carers in trying to understand the nature and severity of the mental health problems that their clients might be experiencing. Put simply, most mental health problems can be allocated to one of two broad categories: psychosis and neurosis.

Psychosis

A psychosis is a serious mental health problem in which clients lack insight into their condition and become out of touch with reality. There is a tendency for psychoses to have a progressively deteriorating course, although in the early stages there may be prolonged periods of recovery between episodes. Ultimately, there will be some deterioration in most aspects of the individual's functioning, including personality, cognitive function, emotional experience, social skills, and daily living skills. Psychoses are typically characterised by delusions (false beliefs), hallucinations (false perceptions), and mood changes. It is often difficult to identify an obvious external cause or trigger factor for the problem, and psychoses are unlikely to resolve without intervention. Indeed, some would say that psychoses can never resolve, only that intervention can minimise the effects on the sufferer or control symptoms.

Psychoses may be described as *organic*, where there is a known physiological cause, or *functional*, where the aetiology is uncertain. Examples of organic psychoses are dementia, a progressive and enduring condition, and delirium, a temporary condition that will subside once the underlying cause is identified (e.g. an infection or toxic reaction to medication). Examples of functional psychoses are schizophrenia and affective (mood) disorders.

Neurosis

A neurosis is a condition characterised by anxiety, in which clients remain in touch with reality and retain insight into their problems, even though they may not be able to resolve them. Although neuroses are usually considered less severe than psychoses, nonetheless they can cause significant suffering and distress to clients and those around them, and the personal consequences of suffering from a neurosis should never be underestimated. Neuroses can often be attributed to an obvious trigger factor, such as a loss or an adverse life change, or a stressful event. They will often resolve without intervention, although intervention can speed up the process of recovery. Examples of neuroses are anxiety, phobias, obsessive–compulsive disorder, and mild depression.

This is a 'rough and ready' classification system only, and there will be many individuals whose mental health problems do not fit neatly into one or other category. Furthermore, there is a range of problems that do not fit neatly into either category, but which have an impact on the mental health of individuals and their families. These include personality disorders, pervasive developmental disorders such as autism, and behavioural problems such as eating disorders or substance misuse. Some of these problems are discussed in Chapter 5. An advantage of such a classification system, however, is that the nomenclature permits a degree of shared understanding between health and social care staff, such that if a psychiatrist describes a client as having, for example, a psychotic episode, there is an instant awareness that this is a serious mental health problem in which the client is likely to have lost some grip on reality; that this problem is unlikely to resolve without a package of interventions, and that it is likely to recur at some future time.

However, it is perfectly possible for an individual to experience both neurotic and psychotic features, and it is sometimes more helpful to think of mental health problems not as falling into discrete categories, but rather as ranging along a continuum of severity. As an example, a person might experience a period of mild depression following an adverse life event, such as the loss of a job. This would normally resolve over time, particularly if the individual was supported by family or friends, and allowed time to come to terms with the new circumstances and decide upon future life directions.

Even following a major loss such as bereavement, it is usual for individuals to begin to pick up the pieces of their life and to adjust to the loss within a reasonable period of time, usually between 1 and 2 years. However, the depression may not resolve within the expected parameters; it may become so prolonged and severe that it is incapacitating to the individual, and begins to affect major areas of functioning and physical health. It may then be suspected that the person is experiencing a more serious depression, which might be described as moderate or severe. The more severe the depression, the more likely the individual will be to display psychotic features such as delusions and thought disorder. It may be, then, that the loss experience was not the direct cause, but rather the trigger factor for an underlying biochemical predisposition to a psychotic mood disorder. What matters to the client, however, is not whether they have a 'psychotic' or a 'neurotic' depression, but rather the effect of the depression upon their daily life and experience, and this will be unique for each individual.

For this reason, the use of the psychosis–neurosis classification system is less frequently used than in the past. Nonetheless, it remains helpful to practitioners and carers from a range of disciplines to have some form of shared understanding about the nature of the problems which clients are experiencing. The ICD-10 classification system (World Health Organization 1992) currently used in the UK offers a more detailed framework for such shared understanding.

ICD-10 provides 11 categories into which mental health problems may be organised, and it is upon ICD-10 that the DC-LD classification system (Royal College of Psychiatrists 2001), designed for use with adults with moderate to profound learning disabilities, is based. This chapter considers four of the ICD-10 categories that also appear in DC-LD, with other categories being considered in Chapter 5. Below we discuss:

- mood (affective) disorders
- neurotic and stress-related disorders
- psychotic disorders/schizophrenia
- organic disorders/dementias.

In each case, there is a consideration of how these problems might impact on the life of people with learning disabilities, their families and carers.

MOOD (AFFECTIVE) DISORDERS

The term 'affect' refers to a transient observed expression of emotion (Bloye & Davies 1999), and is often used synonymously with the word 'mood'. Mood disorders are therefore sometimes referred to as 'affective disorders', and exist when an individual's mood is abnormally depressed or elated. The most common mood disorder is *depression*, a low mood state, but some people suffer from *mania* or *hypomania*, where the mood is abnormally elevated. Mania is an extreme and dramatic elevation of mood, and is somewhat rare, but hypomania, a less extreme form, is seen more frequently. Other mood disorders include dysthymia and cyclothymia (see later in this chapter for a description of these problems).

It is thought that depression and mania are two contrasting presentations of the same disorder, with the most extreme forms represented as opposite poles on a continuum ranging from severe depression to mania. People who experience episodes of both depression and mania or hypomania are said to suffer from *bipolar disorder* (in the past, this was referred to as manic-depressive illness), while those who predominantly experience episodes of depression are said to suffer from *recurrent* or *unipolar depression*. Episodes of mania or hypomania alone do occur, but most clients presenting with mania do eventually go on to develop depression (Gelder et al 1999).

Depression

Depression signifies a mood state that is outside the range of normal mood, either in duration or severity, or both. It is important to distinguish depression from the normal changes in mood experienced by everyone. People may say that they feel depressed, for example, when what they are describing is ordinary sadness or unhappiness. Even when there has been a major precipitating factor or loss, such as bereavement, the grief reactions and low mood that follow are normal and will usually resolve in time. They should not be considered as depression.

Equally, depression may manifest itself in physical symptoms, such as headache or fatigue, which individuals may not recognise or describe as depression, and for which they may therefore not seek or receive appropriate help. In the UK, national interest in depression was stimulated in the 1980s when it was suggested that much depression in the general population was not properly recognised in primary care and therefore did not receive appropriate treatment. This contributed to the development of the 'Defeat Depression' campaign (Royal College of Psychiatrists and Royal College of General Practitioners 1992), a 5-year campaign to emphasise, particularly to GPs, that depression is a common, recognisable, and treatable problem, and that the prognosis for someone with depression is good, even though the condition tends to be recurrent.

It should be noted that depression, particularly in its milder forms, is often accompanied by anxiety, and in this case may be referred to as a 'mixed' disorder. Anxiety in its own right is described later in this chapter.

Prevalence and risk factors for depression

Depression is very common. Around 18% of people are likely to experience an episode of depression at some time in their life, and women are twice as likely as men to experience depression (Bloye & Davies 1999). Many risk factors have been identified, including being aged from late 20s onwards, a member of the working class social group, and living alone. For females, being married or cohabiting with young children, and for men, being unmarried, are risk factors.

Causes of depression

What causes depression? The 'stress–vulnerability' model (Zubin & Spring 1997), originally used to explain the onset of schizophrenia, is helpful in explaining the interaction between existing vulnerability factors in the individual and external life events or stress factors. If exposed to a range of vulnerability factors, the individual might be particularly predisposed to experience depression, but that predisposition may only be precipitated, and a depression activated, when the individual experiences an adverse life event or stress factor.

Vulnerability or predisposing factors

Physical predisposing factors.   There is evidence from population and family studies to suggest that some people inherit a genetic predisposition to depression. Equally, there is evidence that neurochemical factors play a part, and in particular, the neurotransmitters noradrenaline and serotonin are reduced in people with depression.

Social predisposing factors.   In their classic sociological study, Brown & Harris (1978) identified a range of social factors that might predispose people (and women in particular) to depression. These included the lack of an intimate, confiding relationship, being a member of a lower social class, and not having employment outside the home. They also identified the loss of a mother before the age of 11 as a predisposing factor, a theme identified by the psychiatrist John Bowlby during the 1950s and 1960s. In his theory of attachment, Bowlby showed that if attachment to a primary caregiver (often the mother) in the early years of a child's life did not develop securely or was disrupted through separation or deprivation, then that child might have a susceptibility to mental health problems such as depression in adult life (Bowlby 1953).

Several other theories relate to the degree of control that individuals believe that they have over their life and experiences. Seligman (1975), for example, in his theory of learned helplessness, suggested that when people feel that events are happening that are beyond their control, and particularly when attempts to cope with these events seem to fail, then they become helpless in the face of future adverse events. There is a sense of inevitability about their becoming depressed in the face of external stress factors. Equally, Heider's (1958) attribution theory proposed that humans constantly strive to make sense of the world around them and to determine the causes of events in their life. If we believe that the cause of an event lies within ourselves (dispositional attribution), then we are likely also to believe that we have control over that event. If, however, we believe that the cause lies outside ourselves (situational attribution), then we may feel that a solution is out of our hands, and we may become helpless and depressed.

Take, for example, the experience of Jason, introduced in Chapter 2, who lost the job he had held successfully for some time. If he believed that the reason for this was because he had become unreliable, he would know that the solution to this lay within himself. If, however, he believed that he had lost his job because the manager did not like him, then no amount of personal effort could alter this situation, even if his belief was unfounded. It is thought that people who make dispositional rather than situational attributions in relation to their own experiences will better resist depression, or recover from it more effectively if it occurs.

Stress factors

Against the backdrop of these vulnerability factors, which predispose some people to experience depression, what is important is how external events are perceived by the individual, as this will determine whether or not someone becomes depressed. Even when vulnerability factors are present, a vulnerable individual will not necessarily become depressed without the impact of a trigger or stress factor, such as a major life event or a loss experience, which the individual perceives as significant. Sometimes an individual appears to be coping well with a range of stress factors and then succumbs to depression in the light of an apparently trivial event. The phrase 'the straw that broke the camel's back' is apt in describing this experience.

Secondary depression

It should be noted that some physical illnesses are associated with depression; for example, neurological disorders such as multiple sclerosis and Parkinson's disease; endocrine disorders such as hypothyroidism; and some disabling illnesses such as rheumatoid arthritis. Additionally, some prescription and illicit drugs can produce symptoms of depression. Hence it is particularly important that physical illnesses are ruled out before a diagnosis of depression is made.

Symptoms of depression

Today, doctors will aim to distinguish between mild, moderate and severe depression when diagnosing and treating depression. The core symptom of all degrees of depression, however, is a persistently low mood. Normally there will, in addition, be reduced motor activity and broad negative beliefs, such as 'I'm useless', or 'Things will never improve'. In order for a medical diagnosis of depression to be made, not only must other potential problems (such as those mentioned above in secondary depression) be ruled out, but also a range of other symptoms must be present. These may include physical, emotional, behavioural, and cognitive symptoms.

Physical symptoms.   These are often the first indication of problems. Fatigue, sleep changes, loss of energy, appetite and weight changes are all common. Specifically, in relation to sleep, although individuals may have little difficulty in getting off to sleep, they will routinely wake in the early hours of the morning and then be unable to return to sleep. In relation to appetite, although it is most usual for appetite loss and consequent weight loss to occur, over-eating and consequent weight gain is not uncommon.

Emotional symptoms.   Diurnal mood variation is common, meaning that the low mood may occur or be most pronounced at a specific time of day, often the early morning, and is thus associated with early morning waking. Loss of interest and pleasure in usual activities, a sense of anxiety, and irritability, are all common emotional experiences.

Behavioural symptoms.   Associated with loss of interest in activities, the individual will commonly withdraw from everyday social situations. Some people may experience psychomotor retardation, i.e. a slowing down of movements, speech, and gestures. Alternatively, some people will appear agitated and find it difficult to settle.

Cognitive symptoms.   Commonly, people with depression will experience loss of concentration, negative thoughts, low self-esteem, guilt, hopelessness, and sometimes suicidal thoughts. In severe depression thoughts may be distorted such that clients have delusional ideas, often hypochondriacal or persecutory in nature. They may, for example, erroneously believe that they are suffering from a terminal illness, or that others are trying to kill them.

Depression in people with learning disabilities

As with many other mental health problems, mood disorders – and particularly depression – often go unrecognised in people with learning disabilities, despite the fact that they are considered to be at high risk of developing depression. While prevalence rates remain unclear, it is estimated that each year between 3% and 8% of people with learning disabilities will experience depression (Clarke 1999), and much higher rates have been reported. Although there are relatively few data available, it seems that depression occurs particularly commonly in people with Down's syndrome, with some studies reporting three times the incidence of depression in people with learning disabilities of other aetiologies (Cooper et al 1992, Cooper & Collacott 1994, Khan et al 2002, Myers 1999), so this client group may warrant specific attention by carers in identifying early signs of depression.

Vulnerability factors

People with learning disabilities are likely to share the same range of vulnerability factors as the general population. However, as discussed in Chapter 2, many are likely to have experienced significantly more losses and changes, and in some cases abuse and exploitation, in their life, and to experience low self-esteem, lack of social support, lack of control, poor coping skills, and life in less than ideal environments. Specific risk factors such as poor socioeconomic status, vulnerability to abuse, multiple life events, physical health problems, epilepsy, and inappropriate medication have also been identified (Department of Health 1995). It is therefore extremely likely that in the face of a life event, change or stressful situation, depression will be activated, and this is even more likely when changes have been major and frequent. Such life events may, to outward appearances, appear minor, but to the individual, they can be extremely distressing – the 'last straw' phenomenon is just as applicable to people with learning disabilities as to those without.

Assessing depression in people with learning disabilities

Given the high prevalence rates and wide range of vulnerability factors predisposing a person with learning disabilities to develop depression or other mood disorders, how can we recognise the signs of depression in this client group? Regardless of the level of learning disability, common manifestations include sleep disturbance and depressed mood. Indeed, for those people with mild learning disabilities, the presentation of depression will be much as it is for the general population. However, for those people with a moderate disability, the features of weight loss, self-injurious behaviour, reduced communication, a sad, immobile facial expression, and social isolation may be particularly pronounced (Marston et al 1997, Myers 1999). If they are able to verbalise, clients may express ideas of worthlessness (Myers 1999).

For people with severe or profound learning disabilities, existing behaviour problems may become more pronounced, or new behaviours introduced, such as vomiting, incontinence, or smearing of faeces. Additionally, spontaneous crying, screaming, temper tantrums, irritability, anger, self-injurious and aggressive behaviour towards people or objects, excessive sleeping, and loss of skills may be indicative of depression, rather than the more usual depressive symptoms.

These expressions of depression, which increase with increasing levels of disability, have been described as *behavioural depressive equivalents* (Marston et al 1997, Sovner & Lowry 1990), and carers need to become attuned to the potentially wide range of manifestations of depression in their clients. For these clients, it may be possible to observe changes in appearance such as a stooped posture, poor eye contact, and slow movements (Deb et al 2001).

For a diagnosis of depression to be made for a person with learning disabilities, based on DC-LD criteria, a depressed or irritable mood, together with loss of interest, reduction in self-care, social withdrawal, or reduction in communication, will have been present on most days for at least 2 weeks. In addition, four out of a list of nine further symptoms must be present, including tearfulness, distractibility, lethargy, appetite disturbance, and sleep disturbance. These symptoms must represent a change from the person's previous functioning. Assessment must always take into account the risk of self-harm and self-neglect.

Dysthymia and cyclothymia

The term dysthymia was coined in the mid-19th century to describe a poorly understood protracted mood state. More recently, it has been described as a chronically depressed mood, occurring on most days and for most of the day, lasting for at least a year (Masi et al 1999). In other words, while its presentation is likely to mimic depression (Jancar & Gunaratne 1994), the problem is more to do with duration than severity. The prevalence rate for dysthymia in the general population is thought to be around 3%, so in common with most other mental health problems, the prevalence may be higher for people with learning disabilities, and it may often go unreported. In people with learning disabilities, dysthymia may occur following a stressful event, particularly where this involves a loss of some sort.

Whereas dysthymia is a persistently low mood state, in cyclothymia there are recurrent changes of mood, alternating between low mood and mild elation. Some people are described as having a cyclothymic personality. As with dysthymia, cyclothymia is relatively enduring. There is, however, little research evidence available relating to dysthymia and cyclothymia in people with learning disabilities.

Suicide and attempted suicide

The most significant risk factor associated with depression is suicide or attempted suicide, and, *in all cases*, people with depression should be considered to be at risk. In the UK, the severity of the problem has been confirmed through the establishment of targets for the reduction in the number of deaths from suicide (Department of Health 1992, 1999).

While every individual's needs are unique, there is a range of risk factors for suicide that may assist in predicting the likelihood of someone attempting to kill themselves, including:

- having a mental health problem (notably depression, but also schizophrenia)
- a history of alcohol or drug misuse
- poor physical health
- living alone or being homeless
- unemployment.

Furthermore, men are far more likely than women to kill themselves, often employing violent means such as hanging or jumping from high buildings. While older people (75+) have the highest rates of suicide overall, rates for men in the 25–44 age group have risen in recent years. The risk of suicide increases when people have made at least one previous attempt, and/or have a specific plan in mind, particularly if this includes violent means.

It should, however, be noted that risk factors for suicide are not the same for people who deliberately self-harm. In this case, individuals are likely to be young females who predominantly use self-poisoning (drug overdose) as the means of harming themselves. We discuss self-harm more fully in Chapter 5.

Strategies aimed at the reduction of suicide include early recognition of those at high risk, supporting those at risk, and improved education strategies.

Suicide and people with learning disabilities

Suicide is rarely reported in people with learning disabilities, and certainly people with severe or profound levels of disability have traditionally been thought incapable of suicidal intent (Ballinger 1997). Lack of reporting may simply reflect the fact that people with learning disabilities have normally been excluded from epidemiological studies. However, it cannot be assumed that incidences of sudden death are not, in fact, the result of successful suicide attempts. Equally, self-injurious behaviour should be considered as having a potential suicidal intent and not be dismissed as behaviour congruent with the learning disability (an example of diagnostic overshadowing, discussed in Chapters 1 and 3). Although people with Down's syndrome are at higher risk of depression than other people with learning disabilities, it appears that they are much less likely to display suicidal behaviour (Pary et al 1997). Nonetheless, suicide must always be considered, and risk factors identified, whenever a client with learning disabilities is found to be suffering from depression.

Bipolar disorder

This is a recurrent, major mood disorder, in which mood diverges from normal to one or other of the poles of hypomania/mania or depression, often with periods of stable mood in between. Bipolar disorder is much less common than depression alone, with around 1% of the population thought to suffer, and there is no difference in prevalence rates between males and females. A family history of bipolar disorder is often found, and current research is beginning to identify specific genes that may be responsible.

The features of depression described above are the same for both bipolar affective disorder and recurrent depressive disorder. The features of hypomania/mania are described below.

Hypomania/mania

In hypomania or mania, clients experience an elevated mood, and an increase in energy, but at the same time, irritability. They may be over-talkative, and express irresponsible or reckless ideas, which they may attempt to carry out, such as giving away money or belongings, or placing themselves in dangerous situations. They may express grandiose delusions, such as believing they are very wealthy or related to royalty, or flights of ideas, where their conversation appears to jump from topic to topic at a rapid pace. Only the most attentive listener will be able to follow the flow of ideas and discern the tenuous links between them, which are sometimes at the level of rhyming words and plays on words. Concentration will be poor, and there will be a decreased need for sleep. Although they may feel 'on top of the world', they are actually at great risk of causing harm to themselves or other people.

Bipolar disorder in people with learning disabilities

Mixed affective episodes (periods of mania or hypomania alternating with periods of depression) seem to be more common in people with learning disabilities than in the general population, and when they do occur, they tend to be 'rapid-cycling'. This means that there is a quick alternation between depressed and elevated mood, with at least four or more mood episodes per year, but mood changes can occur as frequently as every few hours or even minutes. In other respects, signs and symptoms will resemble those in the general population (Myers 1999). Although depression is common in people with Down's syndrome, they are less likely to experience bipolar disorder than other people with learning disabilities, and this may be due to protective genetic factors (Craddock & Owen 1994).

Assessing hypomania in people with learning disabilities

As with the general population, people with learning disabilities who experience episodes of hypomania or mania are likely to have an increase in motor activity. However, they are perhaps more likely to be irritable or aggressive than euphoric (Deb et al 2001, Vitiello et al 1989). It is possible to identify mania even in people with severe and profound levels of disability as many symptoms can be observed directly or can be ascertained from carers (Deb et al 2001). For a diagnosis to be made, according to DC-LD criteria, clients must have had an abnormally elated, expansive, or irritable mood for at least a week, and in addition must demonstrate three out of a list of nine further symptoms. These include increased talkativeness, reduced sleep, reckless behaviour, and an increase in self-esteem expressed, for example, by grandiose ideas, such as 'I've been invited to the palace to have dinner with the Queen'. It is particularly important, during manic episodes, that attention is paid to clients' physical needs, as they will be far too busy and active to bother to eat, sleep, or take care of their personal hygiene.

NEUROTIC AND STRESS-RELATED DISORDERS

There are several manifestations of neurotic and stress-related problems, the most frequently occurring being generalised anxiety disorder, obsessive–compulsive disorder, and phobias.

Generalised anxiety disorder

Everyone suffers from anxiety from time to time. It is a normal, adaptive response to threat, change, stress, or confusion. It is an emotional and physiological state that anticipates real or imagined threat, and prepares the body to confront and deal with it ('fight') or avoid it ('flight'). A little anxiety can even be considered necessary to enhance physical or intellectual performance, for example when one has to excel in a sporting arena, take an examination, or give a performance on the stage. Most people will, from time to time, feel things 'getting on top of them', and question their ability to cope, but can normally do so when they are able to draw on existing coping strategies or support systems.

However, anxiety can be considered a problem or a disorder when it occurs in situations that most people would normally handle easily, or when it interferes with everyday activities. This might be when the anxiety is exaggerated, prolonged, or inappropriate to the situation. Anxiety disorders are very common. Published estimates of prevalence vary, but it is likely that around 5% of the population will experience generalised anxiety each year (Gelder et al 1999).

Anxiety disorders are characterised by a persistent and sometimes overwhelming feeling of apprehension, accompanied by a range of physical and psychological symptoms. Due to the activation of the autonomic nervous system and the release of the hormone adrenaline from the adrenal gland, the initial presentation is often with physical symptoms such as headache or nausea. Other physical symptoms associated with anxiety include dry mouth, muscular tension, sweating, palpitations, dizziness, and hyperventilation. People with anxiety often have difficulty in getting off to sleep, and often find that the time when they are tossing and turning is the time that their fears and worries are at their most severe.

Psychological symptoms include sensitivity to noise, restlessness, a sense of dread or fearful anticipation, repetitive worrying thoughts, and poor concentration.

Anxiety and people with learning disabilities

Anxiety is relatively poorly researched in people with learning disabilities, and yet it is likely to be a common problem that goes unrecognised and untreated (Raghavan 1998), despite the fact that physical symptoms and fearful facial expressions are readily observable. As with the general population, anxiety is a response to an actual or perceived threat or stress. There is some indication that people with learning disabilities respond to stress with higher levels of anxiety than the general population, and that anxiety is also related to low self-esteem. Unfamiliar problem solving tasks seem to induce great anxiety, and it is thought that clients who are or have been institutionalised have a greater degree of fear and anxiety. Could it be that Geoff, introduced in Chapter 1, is suffering from anxiety due to changes in his environment, altered social contacts, and increased expectations from others? Anxiety in people with learning disabilities might manifest itself as restless pacing, irritability, restlessness, destructiveness, physical aggression, or self-injurious behaviour, particularly in those people who are unable to communicate their distress verbally.

Assessing anxiety in people with learning disabilities

For a diagnosis of generalised anxiety disorder, using DC-LD, a range of symptoms must have been observed on most days for at least 6 months. The client must experience tension, worry, or apprehension, either by describing these experiences or demonstrating fear or anxiety through behaviour. Additionally, they must experience at least one of the symptoms of palpitations, sweating, trembling, shaking, or dry mouth. Further, at least three additional symptoms from a list of 12, including restlessness, repeated swallowing, initial insomnia, distractibility, nausea, vomiting, and chest pain, should be present. Many of these features can be directly or indirectly observed by carers (e.g. frequent drinking or thirst might indicate that the client has a dry mouth; nausea might be considered if the client seems to show little interest in food), and should alert the carer to the possibility of anxiety.

Difficulties in identifying anxiety in people with severe and profound learning disabilities have been noted (Matson et al 1997), and while standardised screening tools such as the DASH-II (see Ch. 6) can assist, assessment and diagnosis will rely heavily on the professional judgement and interpretation of carers.

Obsessive–compulsive disorder

This is an anxiety disorder in which the client experiences *obsessions*, which are persistent intrusions of unwelcome thoughts, images, ruminations, or doubts, and at the same time, normally experiences *compulsions*, which are irresistible urges to carry out certain acts or rituals, and which serve the purpose of reducing anxiety. These acts are repetitive and are not in themselves pleasurable, but failure to carry them out will increase anxiety levels. The most common manifestation of compulsive behaviour in the general population is handwashing.

The prevalence of obsessive–compulsive disorder (OCD) in the general population is thought to be around 1%, and depressive symptoms are sometimes present. There are, as with other mental health problems, several theories concerning the cause of OCD. There may be certain predisposing factors including adverse early childhood experiences such as sexual abuse, or observation of adults' obsessional behaviour. There is some evidence for a genetic predisposition, as familial patterns have been noted. Low serotonin levels have been suggested as a causal factor, as have personality factors. There may be an underlying obsessional personality, manifested as perfectionist traits, but it is important to note that people with obsessional personalities are more likely to develop depression than OCD. As with many other problems, the existence of predisposing factors will not necessarily bring about an episode of OCD without a precipitating stress factor.

OCD and learning disabilities

It is difficult to determine accurate prevalence rates of OCD in people with learning disabilities, although they have been reported as high as 3.5% (Vitiello et al 1989), as it may be difficult to distinguish compulsive behaviours from stereotyped behaviours, which are repetitive/rhythmic movements sometimes found in people with severe learning disabilities. Equally, obsessional traits are often seen as features of pervasive developmental disorders such as Asperger syndrome (see Ch. 5).

Unlike in the general population, where handwashing is most common, the most likely manifestation is 'ordering' (e.g. arranging or counting things) (Vitiello et al 1989), and self-injury may be a feature. Whereas the person in the general population with OCD will try at least some of the time to resist carrying out compulsive acts, resistance by people with learning disabilities to compulsions may be minimal or non-existent. However, attempts by others to prevent compulsions may increase anxiety and result in aggression.

Assessing OCD in people with learning disabilities

It may be difficult to assess the presence of OCD in people with learning disabilities, as they may not possess the level of intellectual sophistication required to describe the subjective symptoms and experiences. Furthermore, it is rarely possible to obtain a clear description of obsessions and compulsions as being a product of the client's own mind (Royal College of Psychiatrists 2001). Hence, assessment and diagnosis will rely heavily on observations of repetitive, ritualistic, or excessive behaviour, and in particular on observing the consequences of the behaviour for the individual. For example, does the client appear more relaxed and settled following the carrying out of some apparently purposeless behaviour?

To arrive at a diagnosis, according to DC-LD, symptoms must be present on most days for at least 2 weeks, and these symptoms must be repetitive and excessive, unpleasant or purposeless, and interfere with social or individual functioning. The client may or may not try to resist the compulsions, but interference from others may increase the distress.

Phobias

A phobia is a particular type of anxiety in which the anxiety is focused on a specific object or situation, or on the anticipation of that object or situation. The amount of anxiety is unreasonable or unfounded, and leads to avoidance of the object or situation. There are three main types of phobia:

- *agoraphobia*, in which the client is afraid to be in public or crowded spaces, or to travel using public transport
- *social phobia*, where fear occurs in social settings such as parties, restaurants, or meetings
- *specific phobias*, such as fear of heights, dogs, snakes, or spiders. However, it must be noted that some fears might be considered reasonable in some circumstances; after all, heights can be dangerous and dogs can bite!

Phobias in people with learning disabilities

As a result of a phobia, people with learning disabilities will experience a range of symptoms either when faced with the feared object or situation, or in anticipation of the feared object or situation. Two of the following symptoms (which are similar to the symptoms of generalised anxiety disorder) should be present in order for a diagnosis to be made, including palpitations, sweating, dry mouth, chest pain, restlessness or irritability. In the case of social phobia, the client may be observed to blush, retch, vomit, or have an urgent need to urinate or defecate. Carers noting these signs of anxiety need to be alert to the situations in which they occur in order that appropriate intervention strategies can be implemented.

Other anxiety disorders

These include panic disorder, where the client experiences recurrent sudden onset panic attacks in which there is intense fear; post-traumatic stress disorder (PTSD) occurring some time following a major stressful experience; and dissociative or somatoform disorders, where the client's anxiety is transferred into bodily sensations and symptoms such as convulsions or amnesia. There is no reason to suppose that these forms of anxiety do not occur in people with learning disabilities; in particular, traumatic life experiences such as abuse may make them particularly susceptible to PTSD. However, there is little specific research or evidence in these areas.

Whatever the form or manifestation of anxiety in people with learning disabilities, the aim should be to prevent its occurrence by anticipating and removing likely stressors. This will depend on excellent observation skills on the part of carers.

PSYCHOTIC DISORDERS

As previously mentioned, psychoses can be subdivided into organic disorders, where there is a known physical cause, or functional, where a definite cause has not yet been established. The most significant functional psychosis is schizophrenia.

Schizophrenia

Schizophrenia has been recognised since 1911, and is a disorder of thinking, perception, mood, and behaviour in which the individual loses touch with reality and often experiences impaired function in a range of areas of everyday life, such as communication and daily living skills. It is not, as the lay person often assumes, a 'split personality', whereby the individual can one day be a 'Jekyll' character, and one day a 'Hyde', with neither character being aware of the existence of the other (although this rare form of personality disorder does exist). This common misunderstanding probably arose out of early attempts to explain the condition and the experience for the sufferer as being like the mind 'splitting' or 'fragmenting'.

Around four people in every thousand are thought to suffer from schizophrenia in the general population (Gelder et al 1999), although it seems to be more common in socioeconomically deprived areas. It is particularly common amongst people who are homeless, but whether this is a cause or an effect is unclear.

What causes schizophrenia?

Schizophrenia appears to be caused by a complex interaction between biological and environmental factors. It is likely that there is an inherited biological predisposition for the development of schizophrenia, although specific genes have yet to be identified. Certainly, a child of one or more parents with schizophrenia has a greatly increased risk of developing the condition, but how much this might have to do with the effects of the home environment and role modelling within the home is uncertain. Against this genetic background, it seems that adverse life events may trigger off an episode of schizophrenia (Zubin & Spring 1997). Furthermore, environmental factors (e.g. family disharmony, hostility or over-involvement from family or carers) or social isolation may maintain the condition or contribute to relapse (Johnstone 1999).

The peak age of onset of schizophrenia is late teens to early twenties. Some people will experience only one episode of schizophrenia in their life, while others will recover but later relapse and experience regular recurrences of the problem. Typically, however, it is an enduring, progressive condition with a relapse–remission pattern, and in many cases there is progressive impairment of functioning between episodes.

Symptoms of schizophrenia

There are, broadly, two kinds of symptom in schizophrenia: *positive symptoms* (sometimes referred to as the acute syndrome), which are pathological by their presence, and *negative symptoms* (sometimes referred to as the chronic syndrome), which indicate the loss of a previous level of functioning.

Positive symptoms

These are behaviours and experiences that were not previously part of the individual's functioning. Typically, the client will experience changes in perception (hallucinations), beliefs (delusions), and thinking (thought disorder), together with impairment in insight, such that the client does not recognise that these are manifestations of an illness that requires intervention and treatment.

Hallucinations. These are sensory perceptions that occur in the absence of external stimuli. Any of the five senses can be affected, but auditory hallucinations are the most common. Clients might hear simple or complex sounds or voices. They might hear their own voice talking out loud, or another voice commenting about them and their actions in the third person, using their name or referring to them as he or she, or voices talking to each other about the client. These experiences are often very distressing, and clients may seem distracted or find it difficult to concentrate on a conversation or a task at the same time as they are experiencing these hallucinations.

Delusions. These are persistent, impossible, unshakeable beliefs, that are out of keeping with the client's cultural or religious background, and which are not amenable to evidence or logic. There are different forms of delusion, but the most common delusions in schizophrenia are *persecutory delusions*, where clients believe that someone or something is against them and wishes them harm, and *ideas of reference*, where clients believe that objects or events around them have a personal meaning for them. For example, they might believe that the newsreader on TV is discussing their particular situation. Sometimes clients experience *delusions of control*, whereby they believe that they are being controlled by an external force or power that they are unable to resist.

Thought disorder. Thought disorder can take the form of *thought insertion*, where clients experience thoughts that are not their own being put into their head; *thought withdrawal*, where clients feel that their thoughts are being taken out of their heads; *thought broadcasting*, where they believe that other people have access to their thoughts, perhaps via the media; and *thought echo*. Thought echo is, in effect, a combination of both a thought disorder and an auditory hallucination, in that clients can actually hear their own thoughts out loud. It follows that these thoughts may not be ones that they would normally choose to share with other people, and yet there seems to be little choice in the matter for them. When we consider that the content of our thoughts is one of the few human experiences that is totally private (unless we choose to share our thoughts with other people), we can imagine the distress that these disturbing alterations to thinking can cause.

Negative symptoms

These become more apparent as the condition becomes more enduring in nature. Typically, we would expect to see emotional changes, such as flattened or inappropriate mood and emotions; behavioural changes, such as loss of drive, initiative, and energy; and apathy. Ultimately we might see loss of communication, loss of daily living skills, and complete social withdrawal. At the same time, the client might continue to experience the positive symptoms of hallucinations, delusions, and thought disorder.

Since the 1970s it has been well accepted that the reactions of other people to the symptoms of schizophrenia, and particularly the negative symptoms, can significantly affect the progression and outcome of the illness. In particular, if clients live within a household or environment where there is 'high expressed emotion' (Vaughan & Leff 1976), i.e. where they receive constant criticism and pressure to change their behaviour, then their chances of relapse, even following successful treatment, are greatly increased.

At the present time, it is not possible to 'cure' schizophrenia, but the advent of a range of new drugs, coupled with advances in psychosocial and early interventions designed to address some of the environmental aspects of the illness (see Ch. 7 for more information on these interventions), offer hope that those who suffer from the condition might be enabled to lead fulfilling and worthwhile lives untroubled by the extremely distressing symptoms of hallucinations, delusions, and thought disorders, and not incapacitated by negative symptoms such as apathy.

Schizophrenia and people with learning disabilities

It is thought that around 3% of people with learning disabilities suffer from schizophrenia (Clarke 1999, Deb 2001), which is considerably higher than in the general population. There are a number of subtypes of schizophrenia identified within ICD-10 but it may be difficult, and not necessarily helpful, to distinguish subtypes in an individual with learning disabilities (Royal College of Psychiatrists 2001).

The complex subjective experiences of schizophrenia (thought disorders, perceptual disorders, delusions) are in themselves extremely difficult for clients to convey to other people. Hence it will be even more difficult for carers to identify these experiences occurring in clients with language and communication difficulties, and there is often a delay in assessing schizophrenia in people with learning disabilities. James & Mukherjee (1996), for example, identified a client who had suffered from schizophrenia for 14 years before a diagnosis was made.

While schizophrenia in people with learning disabilities is likely to share the same aetiology as for the general population, there is a lack of clear evidence as to whether the symptoms are the same. Meadows et al (1991) suggested that there is no difference in the symptoms of schizophrenia in people with learning disabilities and in those without, but some differences have been noted that might aid accurate assessment and diagnosis.

In relation to positive symptoms, the content of delusions and hallucinations may reflect the more limited life experiences of people with learning disabilities and thus be less complex in nature (Došen & Day 2001, James & Mukherjee 1996), making them less easy to identify. Also, whereas delusions are normally unshakeable in the general population, people with learning disabilities may be more compliant and feel pressurised into giving 'acceptable' answers when questioned about delusional ideas (Royal College of Psychiatrists 2001). In other words, they may be more easily 'talked out' of their delusions than would people in the general population. Hence we should be looking for their readiness to restate the delusion either voluntarily or when asked about it. Equally, when evidence that might be indicative of delusions, thought disorder, or hallucinations is presented, it is possible that carers will interpret these as everyday misunderstandings (Royal College of Psychiatrists 2001) or as evidence of the linguistic and communication difficulties experienced by some people with learning disabilities (James & Mukherjee 1996). However, it is normally possible to clarify these misunderstandings, which is not the case with fixed delusional ideas or hallucinatory experiences. While people with learning disabilities can experience all types of hallucination, complex hallucinations such as 'running commentary' are uncommon; such individuals are, however, more likely to experience 'third person' auditory hallucinations than any other types.

It is often difficult to distinguish the negative symptoms of schizophrenia from apathy and withdrawal caused by lack of stimulation, poor environment, or over-sedation in people with learning disabilities, particularly if we do not know the clients' previous level of skills and behaviour. A further difficulty is that some people with learning disabilities present with some atypical features such as over-breathing, pseudo-fits, pseudo-paralysis, and gait disturbance (Došen & Day 2001), making the condition even more difficult to identify and diagnose.

Assessing schizophrenia in people with learning disabilities

Given all these difficulties, carers must become skilled at picking up subtle signs, such as clients appearing distracted, not concentrating on a task, seeming to be talking to themselves, or appearing suspicious. Other early indicators for schizophrenia in people with learning disabilities might include odd or unusual behaviour, aggression, or social withdrawal (Myers 1999).

DC-LD (Royal College of Psychiatrists 2001) provides us with a list of open prompt questions that might be useful in understanding clients' experiences. These include: 'Has anything new happened to you?', 'Is anyone against you?' and 'Has anyone been telling you to do bad things?'. Similarly, the PAS-ADD interview (Moss et al 1993; see Ch. 6) provides samples of questions to identify disordered thoughts and perceptions, such as 'Do people know what you are thinking?' and 'Have you ever heard strange noises that no-one else could hear?'.

For a definitive diagnosis of schizophrenia to be made by a psychiatrist one of the four symptoms of:

- third person auditory hallucinations
- hallucinatory voices from a part of the body
- delusions
- any form of thought disorder

must be present on most days for at least 2 weeks. Additionally, delusions or hallucinations which are not congruent with the client's mood should have been in evidence for most of the time during a month. Finally, two out of five further symptoms, including negative symptoms, should be present on most days for at least 2 weeks. It remains the case, however, that it is extremely difficult to identify with any degree of certainty the presence of schizophrenia in people with severe and profound learning disabilities.

Jason, introduced in Chapter 2, is at the lower end of the age group in which schizophrenia is most likely to develop, and is at the higher end of the intellectual abilities scale. We do not have any clear evidence that he is experiencing hallucinations or delusions, although his daydreaming, not responding to requests or instructions, and staring out of his window for long periods of time might offer clues that he is experiencing some alterations in his perceptual processes. Furthermore, his withdrawal from social contacts and employment might alert us to the early presence of negative symptoms, so the onset of schizophrenia should not be ruled out at this stage.

ORGANIC DISORDERS/DEMENTIAS

Organic disorders are psychoses in which organic pathology leads to brain dysfunction. Whereas most organic disorders are progressive and enduring, *delirium* is an acute brain impairment that can result from a range of physical conditions such as infection, alcohol withdrawal, or drug intoxication. Delirium will normally subside once the cause is identified and treated. *Dementia*, however, is a condition normally occurring in older people, in which there is a gradual deterioration in cognitive areas of functioning such as memory, language, and intellect. There will also be changes in mood, behaviour, and personality. One of the early changes experienced by the client is impaired memory, with memory loss being most obvious for recent rather than past events. This may cause considerable distress to the client who is acutely aware of the changes that are taking place, and which prevent, for example, the easy recall of the names of once familiar people, places, or objects. The first signs noticed by carers, however, may be uncharacteristic or inappropriate behaviour, such as aggression, swearing, or sexual disinhibition. As the condition progresses, attention and concentration become impaired, and the client becomes disorientated, initially for time. Eventually, disorientation for place and person will develop. Throughout, the client is likely to be anxious, irritable, or depressed. In the later stages, thinking becomes disturbed, as will be shown through the content and form of the client's speech.

There are several causes of dementia, the most frequently occurring of which is Alzheimer's disease. Other forms are vascular dementia, Lewy body dementia, and Huntington's disease.

Alzheimer's disease

Alzheimer's disease, more properly known as senile dementia of the Alzheimer's type, or SDAT, is likely to account for around half of all dementias (Deb et al 2001). In the general population, up to 5% of adults aged over 65 are likely to suffer, compared with 20% of those over 80 (Gelder et al 1999). In this condition, senile plaques and neurofibrillary tangles develop in the brain. Early symptoms include impairment of new learning, recent memory loss, and disorientation in time and place. Later, the symptoms of aphasia (difficulty in using or comprehending words), apraxia (difficulty in carrying out motor tasks), and agnosia (failure to recognise familiar objects) may appear, as will disorientation for person, whereby clients lose all sense of who they are as individuals. Ultimately, there will be changes in personality and behaviour, and loss of skills.

One of the problems in identifying the presence of Alzheimer's disease is that it has a slow, insidious onset and is often, in the early stages, mistaken for depression. Conversely, depression may be mistakenly identified as dementia, and to complicate matters further, a person with dementia may also be depressed.

Vascular/multi-infarct dementia

The pattern of this type of dementia is sudden onset with step-wise deterioration, normally following a cerebral infarct (stroke). Burst blood vessels lead to localised brain damage, after which the individual may experience a period of stability until another stroke occurs. Symptoms of vascular dementia are fluctuating, with confusion being common. Emotional and personality changes sometimes occur before cognitive defects are evident.

Other causes of dementia

There is a range of other organic conditions that give rise to dementia. These include Lewy body dementia, a progressive illness with a fluctuating course characterised by hallucinations and delusions; Huntington's disease, a rare degenerative disorder which produces choreiform (brief, involuntary, and purposeless) movements of the face, hands and shoulders; and Creutzfeldt–Jakob disease, a rare and rapidly progressive disorder caused by a prion, which is a new type of disease-causing agent. While Creutzfeldt–Jakob disease affects older people, a new variant is thought to be responsible for 'mad cow disease', which has affected some younger people in the UK.

Organic disorders/dementias in people with learning disabilities

As with physical health, the mental health problems of older people with learning disabilities are similar to those of the population of older people as a whole. However, as with all age groups, mental health problems are more common than in the general population (Day & Jancar 1994). Additionally, because the life expectancy of people with learning disabilities has increased over recent years, due to improved health care generally, we are now seeing more age-related mental health problems. For example, people with Down's syndrome are at particular risk of developing Alzheimer's disease. In the 1930s, a person with Down's syndrome might expect to live only to childhood or teenage years, whereas today, many people with Down's syndrome can expect to reach their 50s and 60s or even older. It now seems that everyone with Down's syndrome who lives to be over 40 will develop the characteristic brain changes associated with Alzheimer's disease, even though not all will go on to demonstrate the clinical features of dementia.

The association between dementia and Down's syndrome was first recognised over 100 years ago, when it was noted that defects found in the brains of people with Down's syndrome at post-mortem were virtually indistinguishable from those of people with Alzheimer's disease (McCarthy 1997). This seems to be due to a genetic link between Alzheimer's disease and chromosome 21, and as people with Down's syndrome have an extra chromosome 21, this may explain their increased vulnerability. Estimates of prevalence in people with learning disabilities range from 11 to 22% (Deb et al 2001) rising to 45% (Marler 2000).

Although the subtypes of dementia (such as Alzheimer's disease, vascular dementia, Lewy body dementia, and Huntington's disease) are likely to be experienced by people with learning disabilities, there is little research into the occurrence of these conditions in people with learning disabilities, and it is not always possible to identify the specific type. Hence it may be more useful to refer to the dementia as being 'unspecified' rather than to try to determine the precise form (Royal College of Psychiatrists 2001). DC-LD provides criteria for the assessment of unspecified dementia.

Assessment of dementia in people with learning disabilities

For people with learning disabilities who do not have Down's syndrome, symptoms and stages of dementia, characterised by cognitive deterioration, are very similar to those in the general population. People with Down's syndrome and Alzheimer's disease will show similar symptoms and stages, although at a younger age. Memory loss, other cognitive deterioration, and emotional changes are the key features. Initially, we might notice apathy, withdrawal, daytime sleepiness, confusion at night, and loss of daily living and self-care skills. Later, gait deterioration, myoclonus (a brief, sudden, shock-like muscle contraction), and the onset of seizures are early indicators (McCarthy 1997), associated with a generalised premature ageing process (Došen & Day 2001). The features of aphasia, apraxia, and agnosia that are commonly seen in the general population are often difficult to measure in people with learning disabilities and so are excluded from the DC-LD criteria (Royal College of Psychiatrists 2001).

In order to diagnose dementia, using DC-LD, symptoms must have been present for at least 6 months. Impaired memory must be present, as must impairment of other cognitive abilities, judgement, or thinking, together with reduced emotional control, such that the client might be emotionally labile, irritable, or apathetic.

CONCLUSION

What may be seen from this chapter is that people with learning disabilities can and do suffer from the same forms of mental health problem as the general population. In many cases, the experience and manifestation of those problems is universal, although in some cases there are some manifestations unique to those with learning disabilities, particularly when the degree of disability is severe. It is hoped that with an increased understanding of the range and manifestations of common problems, carers will be better equipped to identify early signs of mental ill health, to facilitate appropriate assessment and referral, and to advocate for appropriate intervention, such that the quality of life of their clients will be improved. Assessment and intervention strategies are discussed in Chapters 6 and 7. In Chapter 5, more specific problems that impact on mental health are discussed.

REFERENCES

American Psychiatric Association 1994 Diagnostic and statistical manual of mental disorders DSM-IV, 4th edn. American Psychiatric Association, Washington
American Psychiatric Association 2000 Diagnostic and statistical manual of mental disorders DSM-IV-TR (Text Revision). American Psychiatric Association, Washington
Ballinger C 1997 Affective disorders. In: Read S (ed) Psychiatry in learning disability. W B Saunders, London, p 216–236

Bloye D, Davies S 1999 Psychiatry. Mosby, London

Bowlby J 1953 Child care and the growth of love. Penguin, Harmondsworth

Brown G W, Harris T 1978 The social origins of depression. Tavistock, London

Clarke D 1999 Functional psychoses in people with mental retardation. In: Bouras N (ed) Psychiatric and behavioural disorders in developmental disabilities. Cambridge University Press, Cambridge, p 188–199

Cooper S-A, Collacott R 1994 Clinical features and diagnostic criteria of depression in Down's syndrome. British Journal of Psychiatry 165: 399–403

Cooper S-A, Collacott R A, McGrother C 1992 Differential rates of psychiatric disorders in adults with Down's syndrome compared to other mentally handicapped adults. British Journal of Psychiatry 161: 671–674

Craddock N, Owen M 1994 Is there an inverse relationship between Down's syndrome and bipolar disorder? Literature review and genetic implications. Journal of Intellectual Disability Research 38: 613–620

Day K, Jancar J 1994 Mental and physical health and ageing in mental handicap: a review. Journal of Intellectual Disability Research 38: 241–256

Deb S 2001 Epidemiology of psychiatric illness in adults with intellectual disability. In: Hamilton-Kirkwood Z, Ahmed S, Deb S et al (eds) Health evidence bulletins – learning disabilities (intellectual disabilities). NHS, Cardiff, p 14–17

Deb S, Matthews T, Holt G et al 2001 Practice guidelines for the assessment and diagnosis of mental health problems in adults with intellectual disability. Pavilion, Brighton

Department of Health 1992 The health of the nation. HMSO, London

Department of Health 1995 The health of the nation: a strategy for people with learning disabilities. HMSO, London

Department of Health 1999 Saving lives: our healthier nation. Stationery Office, London

Došen A, Day K 2001 Epidemiology, etiology, and presentation of mental illness and behavior disorders in persons with mental retardation. In: Došen A, Day K (eds) Treating mental illness and behavior disorders in children and adults with mental retardation. American Psychiatric Press, Washington, p 3–24

Gelder M, Mayou R, Geddes J 1999 Psychiatry, 2nd edn. Oxford University Press, Oxford

Heider F 1958 The psychology of interpersonal relations. Wiley, New York

James D, Mukherjee T 1996 Schizophrenia and learning disability. British Journal of Learning Disabilities 24: 90–94

Jancar J, Gunaratne I 1994 Dysthymia and mental handicap. British Journal of Psychiatry 164: 691–693

Johnstone L 1999 Do families cause 'schizophrenia'? Revisiting a taboo subject. In: Newnes C, Holmes G, Dunn C (eds) This is madness. A critical look at psychiatry and the future of mental health services. PCCS Books, Ross-on-Wye, p 119–134

Khan S, Osinowo T, Pary R 2002 Down syndrome and major depressive disorder: a review. Mental Health Aspects of Developmental Disabilities 5(2): 46–52

Marler R 2000 Service responses to the 'double disability' of Down's syndrome and Alzheimer's disease. In: Astor R, Jeffereys K (eds) Positive initiatives for people with learning difficulties. Macmillan, Basingstoke, p 147–164

Marston G, Perry D, Roy A 1997 Manifestations of depression in people with intellectual disability. Journal of Intellectual Disability Research 41(6): 476–480

Masi G, Mucci M, Favilla L et al 1999 Dysthymic disorder in adolescents with intellectual disability. Journal of Intellectual Disability Research 43(2): 80–87

Matson J, Smiroldo B, Hamilton M et al 1997 Do anxiety disorders exist in persons with severe and profound mental retardation? Research in Developmental Disabilities 18(1): 39–44

McCarthy J M 1997 Ageing and learning disability. In: Read S (ed) Psychiatry in learning disability. W B Saunders, London, p 237–253

Meadows G, Turner T, Campbell L et al 1991 Assessing schizophrenia in adults with mental retardation. A comparative study. British Journal of Psychiatry 158: 103–105

Moss S, Patel P, Prosser H et al 1993 Psychiatric morbidity in older people with moderate and severe learning disability (mental retardation). Part 1: Development and reliability of the patient interview (the PAS-ADD). British Journal of Phychiatry 163: 471–480

Myers B 1999 Psychotic disorders in people with mental retardation: diagnostic and treatment issues. Mental Health Aspects of Developmental Disabilities 2(1): 1–11

Pary R, Strauss D, White J 1997 A population survey of suicide attempts with and without Down syndrome. Down Syndrome Quarterly 2: 12–13

Prout H T, Stromer D 1998 Issues in mental health counselling with persons with mental retardation. Journal of Mental Health Counselling 20(2): 112–121

Raghavan R 1998 Anxiety disorders in people with learning disabilities: a review of the literature. Journal of Learning Disabilities for Nursing, Health and Social Care 2(1): 3–9

Royal College of Psychiatrists 2001 DC-LD (Diagnostic criteria for psychiatric disorders for use with adults with learning disabilities/mental retardation). Gaskell, London

Royal College of Psychiatrists and Royal College of General Practitioners 1992 Defeat depression campaign. RCP & RCGP, London

Seligman M 1975 Helplessness: on depression, development and death. Freeman, San Francisco

Sovner R, Lowry M 1990 A behavioural methodology for diagnosing affective disorders in individuals with mental retardation. Habilitative Mental Healthcare Newsletter 9: 7

Vaughan C, Leff J 1976 The measurement of expressed emotion in the families of psychiatric patients. British Journal of Social and Clinical Psychology 15: 157–165

Vitiello B, Spreat S, Behar D 1989 Obsessive–compulsive disorder in mentally retarded patients. Journal of Nervous and Mental Disease 177: 232–236

World Health Organization 1992 ICD-10: The international statistical classification of diseases and related health problems, 10th revision. WHO, Geneva

Zubin J, Spring B 1997 Vulnerability – a new view of schizophrenia. Journal of Abnormal Psychology 86: 103–126

5

Specific problems and problem behaviours

INTRODUCTION

As we have seen in Chapter 4, the ICD-10 classification system and the DC-LD system, designed for use with adults with moderate to profound learning disabilities, provide us with a clear framework for identifying and understanding the range of mental health problems that may be experienced by people with learning disabilities. In Chapter 4 we discussed some of the more common mental health problems; this chapter will explore some of the less common problems, all of which appear in some form within the DC-LD (Royal College of Psychiatrists 2001) classification system.

This chapter will address a range of conditions that are related to, produce, or mimic mental health problems, including autism, Asperger syndrome, fragile-X syndrome, and Prader–Willi syndrome. As many of these have self-injury as a feature, a separate section will discuss the problem behaviours of self-injury and self-harm. Personality disorders will be explored as they impact upon people with learning disabilities. Finally, there will be a brief discussion relating to people with learning disabilities who offend, as there may be some relationship between mental health problems and offending.

AUTISM

Autism is a very complex condition. It was first reported in 1943 (Kanner & Eisenberg 1956), and is currently described under the broader headings of 'autistic spectrum disorder' or 'pervasive development disorder'. DC-LD (Royal College of Psychiatrists 2001) lists autism but acknowledges that the diagnostic criteria have not changed from those published in ICD-10 (World Health Organization 1992). Prevalence rates for autism vary from study to study; however the Mental Health Foundation (2000) has suggested a figure in the region of 0.3–0.5%. An in-depth discussion of autism is beyond the scope of this chapter, but the aim is to draw the reader's attention to autism and its relationship to mental health problems.

People with autism have difficulties with the 'theory of mind' concept (Baron-Cohen 1989). When we are in conversation with another person, we make the assumption that the other person thinks, and from this assumption we are able to predict, with some degree of accuracy, the relationship between that person's behaviour and thoughts. We use a range of information to do this, including signs from the environment, the person's body language and voice, and our previous experiences. We then pool this information to create a total interpretation of the world around us, from which we make assumptions about the other person's behaviour and its relationship with their thoughts.

Over time, new experiences become incorporated into our existing body of knowledge so that when we are in new situations we can synthesise existing and new information. However, it appears that people with autism perceive individual behaviours and compartmentalise them, and do not incorporate them into their existing body of knowledge. Thus the central characteristic of autism is an inability to draw together information and derive meaning from that information.

The triad of autism

Autism is not a discrete illness; rather it is a cluster of complex features that encapsulate a broad range of problems. These features can change over time; indeed some may disappear while others may increase. The features are referred to as the triad of impairments.

Impairment of social interaction

People with autism can appear aloof and indifferent to other people. Some may show attachment to people they know well but may be indifferent to others. Some children with autism will approach other people but use odd and inappropriate behaviour in so doing.

Impairment of communication

Many children with autism show lack of appreciation of the use of social language and communication. They lack the understanding that language is an instrument for conveying information to and from others. They also lack understanding of non-verbal communication as in gestures and other body language, and they rarely talk about emotions.

Impairment of flexibility of behaviour and thought

Children with autism have an inability to play imaginatively; they cannot use the 'theory of mind' concept. They seem to have a lack of understanding of the purpose of any activity that involves words and their complex associations. They sometimes copy imaginative behaviours that they have seen elsewhere but cannot explain the meaning of the activities. Play is very rigid and stereotypical, and might include behaviours such as flicking the fingers against light, or spinning objects. More complex behaviours include strong attachment to (or obsession with) objects for no apparent reason, and the fascination of routine, rituals, and movement. People with autism often ask questions repeatedly, even when they have been given the answer. They seek sameness and display anxiety when routines are changed in any way, and they sometimes self-injure.

The range of behaviours and problems is broad, and the intensity ranges considerably, as does the ability level of people with autism, hence the overarching concept of 'autistic spectrum disorder'. However, everyone on the spectrum has some degree of impairment within the triad of impairment.

Causes of autism

As yet there is no complete explanation for the cause of autism. It can be viewed as a biological reaction, as a cognitive deficit, or as an emotional disability (Anderson 2003). Originally it was thought that poor parenting skills caused autism, and that it was only associated with middle-class families. Mothers, in particular, who wanted to develop careers, were thought to be 'cold' carers, contributing to the development of the identified behaviours. Fortunately these ideas no longer have any substance, and it is recognised that autism can be found in any type of family setting.

A more recent view is that autism is a genetically transmitted disorder (Le Couteur et al 1995). There are links to fragile-X syndrome, Down's syndrome, and tuberous sclerosis (tuber-like growths on the brain which can lead to learning disabilities). Other biological causes have been suggested, including phenylketonuria (a hereditary but controllable disease that is caused by the lack of a liver enzyme required to digest phenylalanine; if this is not digested then damage to brain tissue will occur, leading to learning disabilities), and other metabolic abnormalities, infections, and diseases such as rubella and postnatal herpes virus. There is currently a suggestion that the triple vaccination against mumps, measles and rubella (MMR) may contribute to the onset of autism, although there is a lack of convincing evidence in this respect (Shattock 1997). More recently, Nasr & Roy (2000) have reported on balanced chromosomal translocation in a study of monozygotic twins with severe learning disabilities, autism, and affective disorder, and while they do not give conclusive evidence that the autism was genetically caused, their research certainly adds to the debate.

Mental health problems in people with autism

Mental health problems can occur as a secondary disorder amongst people suffering from autistic spectrum disorders (Došen & Petry 1994), as they are not immune to the common mental health problems suffered by the general population. As with all mental health problems in people with learning disabilities, it is sometimes difficult to distinguish between the behaviours that are exhibited by a person with autism, and a possible link with mental health problems. For example, Simone, who is 21, has autism, and each morning her mother has to set the table in exactly the same way, the way that Simone demands. If this is not done, Simone throws a tantrum and becomes verbally aggressive towards her mother. Is Simone behaving badly and thus requiring behavioural interventions, or is she suffering from obsessive–compulsive disorder? Many people with autism are very ritualistic and do not want their routines changed. It has also been demonstrated that affective disorders are frequent in people with autism.

Let us now turn to two specific mental health problems linked with autism: depression and schizophrenia.

Autism and depression

As we saw in Chapter 4, depression is a very common problem, in both the general and the learning disabled population. Although there have been no large scale epidemiological studies, clinically based studies suggest that depression is also the most common mental health problem in people with autism (Ghaziuddin et al 2002). In fact Kanner, who originally identified autism, showed that some of the children in his original study had symptoms of altered mood. Although the cause is unclear, it has been suggested that children with autism who suffer from depression are more likely to come from a family with a history of depression, indicating either a genetic or environmental link, or an interaction between the two.

Because people with autism experience difficulty in interpreting both their own and other people's non-verbal communication, and because they have difficulty in communicating emotions, the identification of depression in people with autism can be extremely difficult. Furthermore, diagnostic overshadowing may mean that symptoms of depression go unnoticed, thus delaying appropriate intervention. Often a diagnosis is dependent on the subjective interpretations of the family or carer.

As we saw in Chapter 4, the manifestation of depression in people with learning disabilities can be different from within the general population, and this is certainly true in people with autism. They tend to exhibit heightened autistic behaviours; for example they may drastically increase their obsessive–compulsive behaviours (Ghaziuddin et al 1995).

Autism and schizophrenia

During the early development of knowledge of autism there were strong suggestions that there was a relationship between schizophrenia and autism, and the term 'childhood schizophrenia' was often used to describe children with autism. These children are now adults, and with improved diagnostic facilities and greater understanding of autism, we are now able to challenge the original diagnosis of schizophrenia.

It is true that some of the features of autism can mimic the negative symptoms of schizophrenia. For example, people with autism can be socially withdrawn, show flattened affect, have poverty of speech, and communication problems. Although they rarely display the positive features of schizophrenia, such as hallucinations and delusions, people with high-functioning autism do have a cognitive profile that resembles that of some of the subgroups of schizophrenia (Goldstein et al 2002). It is here again that the issue of diagnostic overshadowing becomes relevant, and we have to ask several questions.

- *Are the similar symptoms an indication of the same underlying problem?* For the past 30 years it has been shown that schizophrenia and autism are two clearly distinct neurodevelopmental disorders. The early view that both disorders manifest different symptoms of the same underlying problem is no longer a viable proposition, although there may be some underlying links (Konstantareas & Hewitt 2001).
- *Does one disorder lead to another?* One particular study in the late 1980s suggested that this might be the case. Clarke et al (1989) reviewed five clients with Asperger syndrome (see below) and autism; four of these went on to develop schizophrenia in later life. However, this small scale case review cannot be taken to suggest that the majority of people with Asperger syndrome or autism will develop schizophrenia, and considerably more research is required.

INTERVENTION

At the root of achieving improvement in the quality of life for an individual with autism, with or without a mental health problem, is the need to develop an early treatment plan. There is no effective physical intervention that can correct autism; hence interventions need to be directed at a psychological level and begin as soon as possible in childhood. Unfortunately, the use of psychotropic medication has in the past been widespread, leading to over-prescribing and the adverse effects of sedation (see Ch. 7), which can inhibit the therapeutic effects of any other intervention that the carer may wish to use.

On a positive note, relaxation therapy has been used successfully in children with autism; Mullins & Christian (2001), for example, reported how they were able to reduce a child's maladaptive behaviour through relaxation therapy, and help him to develop coping strategies that could be generalised across differing settings. There are, however, few studies that examine the treatment of depression or other mental health problems in people with autism, and further research is required.

ASPERGER SYNDROME

Asperger syndrome is an example of a pervasive developmental disorder that shares many characteristics with autism. Hans Asperger identified this condition in 1944, a year after Kanner reported his findings on autism. The children that Asperger studied produced stilted, repetitive speech, and while they were able to form relationships, they were unaware of the social behaviours that supported these relationships.

Asperger syndrome is defined by impairments in social relationships and communication abilities. People with Asperger syndrome also exhibit repetitive behaviours, interests, and activities (Barnhill 2001). They do not appear to be able to understand the unwritten rules used by other people when conducting themselves in their everyday communications. Thus people with Asperger syndrome have major problems in coping with their social interactions and the world around them.

Asperger syndrome appears to have a later onset than autism. This could be because complex relationships are only beginning to be formed once school and teenage years arrive, and when relationships are crucial to development.

There are some obvious similarities between Asperger syndrome and autism. Asperger himself did not view the disorder as a variant of autism, although many people consider Asperger syndrome to be at the higher end of the autistic spectrum, with autism at the lower end in relation to ability and severity. Another view, based on neurobehavioural evidence, is that autism and Asperger syndrome are two distinct conditions; indeed both the DSM-IV (American Psychiatric Association 1994, 2000) and the ICD-10 (World Health Organization 1992) classify them as two separate entities. As we have seen, many people with autism also suffer from learning disabilities. Although Wing (1981) argued strongly that people with Asperger syndrome could have learning disabilities (and this suggestion continues to be researched), the majority of people with Asperger syndrome have average to above average intelligence. Hence DC-LD (Royal College of Psychiatrists 2001) does not include Asperger syndrome within its diagnostic categories.

However, as they have significant problems in generalisation of knowledge and skills and higher levels of thinking, people with Asperger syndrome may experience academic difficulties.

The syndrome was only recognised by the American Psychiatric Association as a pervasive developmental disorder in 1994. There is therefore limited scientific research to aid diagnosis, which has to be founded on the behaviours that the person exhibits. Attempts have been made to produce diagnostic criteria (e.g. Wing 1981), but with the wide range of reported characteristics, such as insistence on sameness, poor concentration, academic difficulties, vulnerability to emotional problems, memory complications, sensory processing problems, motivation and problem solving difficulties, and motor problems (clumsiness), these are difficult to produce. However, there is some agreement that the fundamental characteristics of Asperger syndrome consist of a significant impairment in social relationships to the degree that it affects quality of life, significant deficits in communication, and finally a restricted range of interests or flexibility of thought.

Asperger syndrome may go undiagnosed until early adulthood, and it is at this stage of life that many people who suffer from Asperger syndrome develop depression and anxiety. Some 25 years ago it was estimated that 30% of adults with Asperger syndrome suffered from depression (Wing 1981). More recently Ghaziuddin (1998) has suggested a prevalence rate for depression of 37%.

FRAGILE-X SYNDROME

Fragile-X syndrome is recognised as the most common inherited cause of learning disabilities. The syndrome is called fragile-X as there exists a fragile site at the end of the long arm of the X-chromosome in the lymphocytes of affected people. More boys than girls are affected; mothers who carry the affected gene have a 30–40% chance of having an affected boy and a 15–20% chance of having an affected girl. Often there is a history of learning disabilities or problems of development on the maternal side of the family.

Physical features include a long face, large prominent ears, large jaw, high arched palate, flattened nasal bridge, prominent forehead, microcephaly (abnormally small head) or relative macrocephaly (abnormally large head), epicanthic folds (folds of skin over the eyes), simian creases (a single crease across the palm of the hand), long philtrum (the groove in the upper lip that runs from the top of the lip to the nose), and post-puberty macro-orchidism (enlarged testicles). The full range of intellectual disability can be experienced, with boys tending to be more severely disabled than girls.

Common concerns that parents identify include delays in speech and development, short attention span, hyperactivity, the mouthing of objects, problems with disciplining the child, temper tantrums, self-injurious behaviour, and autistic-like behaviour such as rocking, flapping hands, talking to oneself, poor eye contact, and spinning.

PRADER–WILLI SYNDROME

Prader–Willi syndrome was first identified in 1956 by Prader, Lahbart and Willi. It affects one in 10 000 live births and is a genetic disorder that can affect people in many different ways. There are four possible causes:

- *Imprinting error in chromosome 15*. Imprinting is where a chromosome is marked so that there are differences between maternal and paternal inheritance.
- *Deletion of part of chromosome 15*. Around 60–70% of people with Prader–Willi syndrome have part of chromosome 15, inherited from their father, missing.
- *Both chromosomes inherited from the mother*. In about 25% of cases, Prader–Willi syndrome can be the result of disomy, i.e., when two copies of the same chromosome are inherited from the mother rather than one from each parent.
- *Translocation of chromosome 15*. This is where material has been exchanged between chromosomes.

The clinical picture of Prader–Willi syndrome is complex. At birth the child is usually small and floppy with absent or weak sucking, which warrants admission to a special care baby unit. As the child grows, physical features develop including narrow face, almond-shaped eyes, and small feet, hands, and genitalia. These children often have blond hair and blue eyes. Due to their floppiness and weak muscle tone they are late to sit and walk and often appear small for their age, with difficulties in feeding, and are slow to gain weight in their first year. In the toddler years (1–4) they develop an insatiable desire for food, and begin the process of rapid weight gain that lasts throughout life. Though this can be controlled somewhat by a strict diet, it presents a major problem for families. The weight gain is partly due to the behavioural problem of demanding food or stealing food from any accessible place, and partly due to calorie intake. Because of their weak muscle tone, they are not able to burn up calories during play and other physical activities, and so are prone to weight gain. Scoliosis may occur at any age, but the child is at more risk during puberty, which is often delayed.

Intellectually, the average IQ is 70 with some people having severe learning disabilities and some having an IQ of around 100. A behavioural phenotype has been described which includes sleep abnormalities, perseveration (the habit of continually asking repetitive questions), obsessive–compulsive behaviours, self-mutilation by way of skin picking, and a vulnerability to low mood and psychotic symptoms. Children with Prader–Willi syndrome often have difficulties in carrying out instructions, and repeatedly request reassurance; this may in part be due to auditory problems. They insist on routine and have difficulty in dealing with change; this is often manifested in stubbornness and temper tantrums. As adults these problems persist, weight gain leads to obesity, and life expectancy is short. Few people with Prader–Willi syndrome live to be over the age of 40.

Treatment for people with Prader–Willi syndrome varies in relation to the degree of learning disabilities. Dietary management is indicated, but is often difficult to maintain due to the intensity of the demands made by the client. Medication, behavioural and psychological approaches have all been used to address the mental health problems associated with Prader–Willi syndrome.

LESCH–NYHAN SYNDROME

Lesch–Nyhan syndrome was first described in 1964 by Michael Lesch and William Nyhan in relation to the unusual features and behaviours of two brothers. It is a very rare disease affecting approximately 1 in 800 000 children, and is caused by a defective gene on the long arm of the X chromosome resulting in the lack of an enzyme known as HPRT (hypoxanthine-guanine phosphoribosyltransferase). The condition affects males almost exclusively, as the defective gene is recessive. Females can be carriers, however, and the condition may be either inherited or a gene mutation may take place spontaneously. The condition is devastating, with its main characteristics being severe dystonia (postural disorder), spasticity, speech impairments, renal disease, varying levels of learning disability and, most strikingly, an innate compulsion to self-injure. Lesch–Nyhan syndrome appears to be distributed evenly across race, income, and geographical location. First indications of the condition can be seen at 3–6 months of age, when orange-coloured crystals are found in the child's urine. This is due to an increased amount of uric acid in the urine. The increased uric acid may also cause the formation of sodium urate crystals in the joints, kidneys, and central nervous system, leading to problems with joints, kidney stones, dysphagia (difficulty in swallowing), vomiting, hypotonia (reduced muscle tension), athetosis (involuntary movements), and behavioural problems including self-mutilation, uncontrolled aggressiveness, and compulsive behaviour. The build up of uric acid can cause severe pain, distress, and self-mutilation.

The self-injurious behaviour exhibited is severe. Often lip and cheek biting occur as early features, along with eye gouging, finger biting, and head butting. Some older children have mutilated faces and hands due to constant biting and pulling. As the child gets older, more self-injurious behaviours develop, such as trapping hands in objects, or forcing fingers through spokes in wheelchairs. Aggression is exhibited through spitting, kicking, head butting, and swearing at carers. Some children apologise immediately, indicating that they are aware of their behaviour but are unable to control it. The onset of such behaviours is sudden and violent, whereas in other children with similar behavioural problems, the onset is more likely to be gradual (Hall 2001).

Treatment can appear archaic, in that physical restraints sometimes need to be used. However, there are reports suggesting that properly designed restraints can enable the child to experience a range of positive activities and feel a sense of security (Anderson & Ernst 1994). Pharmacological treatments appear to be ineffective in that they only reduce self-injury for short periods of time. One approach that has shown to be effective is to ignore the behaviours. However, this does carry consequences for carers who may be spat at, kicked, and bitten. Hall (2001) has suggested that control of the environment and levels of social interaction may reduce the frequency of self-injurious behaviour, hence environmental interventions should form a part of any care management approach. Unfortunately, the prognosis for individuals with Lesch–Nyhan disease is poor as there is no effective treatment available, and death in early adulthood is the usual outcome.

CRI DU CHAT SYNDROME

Cri du chat ('cry of the cat') syndrome was first identified in France in the early 1960s by Lejeune. Prevalence rates are currently estimated as 1 in 50 000 live births (Royal College of Psychiatrists 2001). Though not a very respectful term, a cat-like cry is one of the major characteristics of the condition identified in some but not all newborn infants. Originally it was thought that all sufferers would have severe learning disabilities, together with abnormal facial features such as microcephaly (abnormally small head), rounded face, hypotelorism (very close eyes) with downward sloping palpebral fissures (abnormalities of the eye opening), low set ears, broad nasal ridges, and a short neck. It was also thought that sufferers would have restricted language skills and severe psychomotor development problems. These descriptors were challenged in the 1980s and 1990s, however, and it is currently recognised that these features are not present in all cases.

Cri du chat syndrome is now referred to as 5p as it is recognised that the condition is caused by a deletion of chromatin from the short arm of chromosome 5 (Cornish & Bramble 2002). Studies have shown that children with milder conditions tend to have educational difficulties rather than learning disabilities, and may have an IQ within normal ranges. Self-injurious behaviour is very common, including head banging, hitting the head against body parts, and self-biting. Attention deficit and hyperactivity have also been identified as features of 5p.

SELF-INJURY AND SELF-HARM

As we have seen, many of the syndromes giving rise to learning disabilities described in this chapter are associated with self-harm, creating particular challenges for families and carers. However, there are many forms of self-harm that cannot be accounted for by being associated with a specific syndrome.

In the UK, drug overdose is the most common method of inflicting self-harm in the general population, whereas self-inflicted injuries such as cuts to the arms, wrists, and hands account for about 5–15% of hospital admissions. People who self-injure tend to be young, with low self-worth, unstable moods, and difficulties in maintaining relationships. Causes of self-harm usually result from either a mental health problem or negative social experiences.

It is difficult to define self-injurious behaviour due to the very complex nature of the act. It can be described as the deliberate act of damaging one's own tissues without the intention of taking one's life. A simple classification suggested by Favazza & Rosenthal (1993) gives three basic types – major, superficial, and stereotypic:

- a major classification is associated with acute mental health or severe personality problems
- a superficial classification would describe symptomatic features of mental health disorders
- a stereotypic classification is often attributed to people with learning disabilities who have spent long periods in institutional settings.

The final (stereotypic) classification can, however, be misleading. Longitudinal studies have shown that when people with a record of self-injurious behaviours are moved to small group living in the community, they continue to self-injure for many years to come.

A further problem in defining self-injurious behaviour is that it varies from person to person. Because of the problems in actually defining what self-injury is, and the different methods used to identify, research, and classify the behaviour, there is an associated problem of identifying prevalence rates. Emerson et al (1997) estimate a range from 2% to 5%, but that figure can be based only on people who access services, and can therefore be counted.

Self-injury, self-harm, and people with learning disabilities

The most common forms of self-injury exhibited by people with learning disabilities include self-biting, punching and slapping, skin picking, pica (the eating of non-edible material), and head banging. Studies have shown that people who self-injure also exhibit other forms of challenging behaviour (Emerson et al 1997). The consequences of self-injury may have a profound effect on the quality of the client's life. Restrictions may be placed on community living experiences, and physically the individual may develop infections, have physical deformities, loss of eyes, and even limbs. Most treatment regimes tend to be behavioural in focus, and although evidence does suggest that self-injurious behaviour can be reduced, it is not always eliminated.

Causes of self-injury

There are a number of theoretical arguments as to the cause of self-injurious behaviour amongst people with learning disabilities; none has been scientifically confirmed. Behavioural theories suggest that the behaviour is reinforced when rewards are received. In the case of self-injury the behaviour may have happened accidentally but the person received a reward such as attention from a carer; this attention perpetuates more self-injurious behaviour and more attention.

One factor that some people with severe learning disabilities have in common is a lack of social skills and the ability to adapt to their environment, which are crucial to adjustment and normal functioning (Matson et al 2003). Unfortunately, it has also been reported that deficits in this area can lead to problem behaviours including self-harm (Duncan et al 1999).

Self-injury is also associated with the stimulation of neurotransmitters in the brain. For example, over-sensitivity of the dopamine receptor may lead to self-injury. This has been demonstrated in people with Lesch–Nyhan syndrome. Raised endorphin levels have also been associated with self-injury. A chemical elevation of the pain threshold can lead to the maintenance of self-injury once the behaviour has shown to produce desired responses from carers.

As we have seen, many syndromes discussed in this chapter identify self-injury as a significant feature. Other syndromes in which there are high rates of self-injury include Cornelia de Lange syndrome, also known as Amsterdam dwarfism, where the person has small feet and hands, microcephaly, facial hair, slanting eyes, irregular teeth, and learning disabilities; and Tourette's syndrome, a neurological disorder characterised by tics, which are repetitious, involuntary, rapid, sudden movements. People with Tourette's syndrome often display self-injurious behaviours such as head banging or hitting themselves on the lips or tongue.

Self-injurious behaviour in people with learning disabilities is found at all ages, and assessment and intervention should be carried out as soon as possible. Assessment tools such as the Behaviour Problems Inventory are available to assist in this process (Rojahn et al 2002). Treatment of self-injury in people with learning disabilities has in the past been largely restricted to pharmacological interventions to the extent that clients were given high doses of medication in order to reduce their activity. More recently, treatment programmes using behavioural approaches have been used, though they are not always successful.

PERSONALITY DISORDER

As individuals we all have our own unique personality profile which makes us different from every other person. We all have our own set of values, beliefs, and attitudes, enabling us to make judgements about other people, situations, and the meaning of life. Our personalities are formed from the interaction between genetic and environmental factors and life experiences. So when does our individuality or our personality become a problem or a disorder? Personality disorders can be seen as enduring and inflexible ways of living that encompass all areas of functioning, and which can create problems either for the individual or more often for those within their social network. Within the general population, a range of personality disorders are identified in both ICD-10 (World Health Organization 1992) and DSM-IV (American Psychiatric Association 1994, 2000), which can be sum-marised under the following broad groupings (Gelder et al 1999, Lemma 1996):

- *Anxious and moody personalities.* People in this group are constantly anxious and fearful about their everyday life. Others may have a depressed mood or have fluctuating moods (cyclothymic personality). People who have obsessive–compulsive personality traits, or who are indecisive or obstinate, also fall into this grouping.
- *Sensitive and suspicious personalities.* In this group, personalities can be described as paranoid, schizoid or schizotypal. People in this group tend to be mistrusting and suspicious, and can be seen by others as being irritable and touchy.
- *Dramatic and impulsive personalities.* People in this group like to be at the centre of attention and dramatise their problems. They can be very enthusiastic but soon lose the motivation to continue with activities they have started. They tend to be unaware of the impact that they have on others. Some act impulsively, which sometimes results in self-harm, and some have excessive admiration for themselves (narcissistic personality), although this may mask low self-esteem.
- *Aggressive and antisocial personalities.* Many years ago these people were referred to as psychopaths, but today when this personality trait is severe it is referred to as antisocial personality disorder. People in this group act on impulse without any feelings of guilt or consideration for others. They have a low tolerance for frustration and may become violent if thwarted. They show little concern for other people's emotions, and are superficial in their relationships, which often break

down. They tend to have family problems, often commit criminal offences, and do not learn from their experiences.

Personality disorder and people with learning disabilities

When we begin to examine the personalities of people with learning disabilities, there are several factors that should be considered before we begin to assess for personality disorder. We should consider the social environment in which the person is functioning; this will have an impact on their personality. Clients who have lived in long stay institutions will have gained different life experiences compared with their counterparts who have been functioning within a family network. The environment in which people live has an impact on behaviour. Just because a client constantly seeks attention from the home leader or their carer does not mean that they have a dramatic or impulsive personality; it could be that they just cannot communicate their wishes, and the way in which people with learning disabilities respond to reinforcers will shape their personality.

Many people enjoy a degree of success in their life, be it academically, in acquiring a skill, or within relationships; unfortunately this is not always the case in people with learning disabilities, especially when this is severe. This can lead to a low expectancy of success, and a life history of failure to succeed could lead to them becoming anxious or moody, but this does not mean that they have a personality disorder. Finally, people with learning disabilities who exhibit violent and aggressive behaviours need not necessarily have antisocial personalities; this may be the only way they can communicate their needs.

Studies report a range of prevalence rates for personality disorder in people with learning disabilities. In the mid 1980s it was shown that there was a greater likelihood that people living in long stay institutions would have personality disorders and that prevalence rates were in the region of 22% (Reid & Ballinger 1987). Other studies have suggested rates ranging from 3% to 90%, demonstrating that there are many difficulties in identifying and therefore diagnosing and treating people with learning disabilities and a personality disorder. Difficulties arise in the communication levels of clients that allow them to inform us of their thoughts and ideas. Again diagnostic overshadowing informs us that we need to be careful when suggesting that a person has a personality disorder when in fact it could also be part of their learning disability or a mental health problem.

There are no validated tools for measuring personality disorder in people with learning disabilities, although tools for the general population such as the Standardised Assessment of Personality (Mann et al 1981) have been used (Deb et al 2001). DC-LD suggests that personality disorder should not be diagnosed in people with learning disabilities under the age of 21, to allow for continued development of the personality, and that a diagnosis is avoided in people with severe and profound disabilities. It further recommends that certain subcategories of personality disorder – particularly schizoid, dependent and anxious – are not used as there are difficulties in making differential diagnoses in these categories. In some cases it may only be possible to make a diagnosis of 'personality disorder: unspecified'. Naik et al (2002) suggest that in day-to-day clinical practice, a diagnosis of personality disorder is likely only to be considered for a small number of clients with reasonable cognitive and verbal abilities.

PEOPLE WITH LEARNING DISABILITIES WHO OFFEND

The literature regarding people with learning disabilities who offend is minimal even though this group of people is not immune from the criminal justice system, and services are increasingly being asked to take referrals in such cases (McBrien 2003). Several studies have attempted to give prevalence rates, but it is difficult to give accurate figures as much of the research has varied in sample size, source of sample, and access to judicial services. There are also other difficulties as the police have the right not to press charges, so if a person with learning disabilities has committed an offence they still may not be recorded as offending. Most people with learning disabilities who offend are in the mild to moderate intellectual ability range and, as in the general population, tend to be male. What is interesting, however, is that there is an unusually large proportion of people from ethnic minority groups, although as yet the reasons for this are not known. In Britain people with learning disabilities can be found to be unfit to plead, and if a person is classified as having a mental disorder or mental impairment under the Mental Health Act (1983), then these people can be referred to hospitals for treatment rather than be sent to a prison for custodial punishment. What is of note is that a small number of longitudinal studies demonstrate that people with learning disabilities who have been admitted to mental health services have an increased risk of offending (for a more detailed account see Murphy & Mason 1999), but it is difficult to determine whether mental health problems lead to offending, or vice versa, or indeed whether the relationship is coincidental.

McBrien's (2003) literature review has outlined methodological problems, not only in identifying which offenders have learning disabilities, but also which people with learning disabilities offend, and considerably more research needs to be conducted to ascertain accurate prevalence rates and develop appropriate interventions and services.

CASE STUDY AND CONCLUSION

In this chapter we have introduced a range of problems that might be experienced by people with learning disabilities that can be associated with, mimic, or give rise to mental health problems. It is important that carers have an understanding of such problems in order to make informed needs assessments and to select appropriate interventions. The case study of David, below, illustrates some of the key issues.

Case study: David

David, 28, has moderate learning disabilities. Physically he is a tall gentleman, of average weight for his height, and he is ambulant although he has a slight limp. He lives in a small group home in the centre of town and accesses a local college for clients of similar ability. At home he often sits alone and does not seem to like the company of other people. When his parents come to visit he will often move away from them; they find this distressing but maintain as much contact with him as he permits. He has no verbal skills but is able to communicate using modified Makaton signs that he and the care staff have developed. Two months ago the owners of the home changed, and a new manager has been employed. David tends to self-injure on a daily basis; his main problem is that he rubs his eyes and prods at them until they bleed. Currently his eyes are very sore.

Exercise

- What do you think is happening with David, in terms of learning disabilities and mental health problems?
- How might your knowledge of specific conditions help you to understand David's situation?
- As the new manager of his home, how could you begin to improve the quality of David's life?
- Who should be involved in developing a care package for David?

There is a range of mental health problems that David could be experiencing, including anxiety, depression, obsessive–compulsive disorder, schizophrenia, and self-harm. His self-injurious behaviour might lead us to suspect that he has one of the specific syndromes described in this chapter, although if this is the case, we are likely to have known about it for a long time. As a carer it is important not to allow assumptions to drive care planning, as David may not have any of these problems. You may have concluded that carrying out a functional analysis might identify the stimuli for David's behaviour, and it will be important to take a detailed history from his records, his family, and care staff. Assessment tools such as the Behaviour Problems Inventory (Rojahn et al 2002) may be helpful here. His daily activities may have to be reviewed to see what benefit he is getting from them and whether they could be improved.

The identification of any specific mental health problem may help to determine appropriate interventions for David, and spending time with him in order to develop a therapeutic relationship upon which assessment can be based may uncover possibilities not previously considered.

Finally, there are clearly some new difficulties affecting David's relationship with his parents, and they may be just as helpful, if not more so, than professional carers in determining and helping to identify these difficulties and respond to his needs.

In Chapter 6, we begin to explore some of the ways in which assessment of mental health problems can be carried out, with specific reference to diagnostic criteria and assessment tools.

REFERENCES

American Psychiatric Association 1994 Diagnostic and statistical manual of mental disorders DSM-IV, 4th edn. American Psychiatric Association, Washington

American Psychiatric Association 2000 Diagnostic and statistical manual of mental disorders DSM-IV-TR (Text Revision). American Psychiatric Association, Washington

Anderson L T, Ernst M 1994 Self-injury in Lesch–Nyhan disease. Journal of Autism and Developmental Disorders 24: 67–81

Anderson M 2003 Autistic spectrum disorder. In: Gates B (ed) Learning disabilities: towards inclusion, 4th edn. Churchill Livingstone, London, p 183–204

Barnhill G P 2001 What is Asperger syndrome? Interventions in School and Clinic 36(5): 259–265

Baron-Cohen S 1989 The autistic child's theory of mind: a case of specific developmental delay. Journal of Child Psychology and Psychiatry 30: 285–297

Clarke D J, Littlejohns C S, Gorbett J A et al 1989 Pervasive developmental disorders and psychosis in adult life. British Journal of Psychiatry 155: 692–699

Cornish K, Bramble A 2002 Cri-du-chat syndrome: genotype–phenotype correlations and recommendations for clinical management. Developmental Medicine and Child Neurology 44: 494–497

Deb S, Matthews T, Holt G et al 2001 Practice guidelines for the assessment and diagnosis of mental health problems in adults with intellectual disability. Pavilion, Brighton

Došen A, Petry D 1994 Psychiatric and emotional adjustment of individuals with mental retardation. Current Opinion in Psychiatry 7: 387–391

Duncan D, Matson J L, Bamburg J W et al 1999 The relationship of self-injurious behaviour and aggression to social skills in persons with severe and profound learning disabilities. Research in Developmental Disabilities 20: 441–448

Emerson E, Alborz A, Reeves D et al 1997 The HARC challenging behaviour project. Report 2: The prevalence of challenging behaviour. Hester Adrian Research Centre, University of Manchester

Favazza A, Rosenthal R 1993 Diagnostic issues in self-mutilation. Hospital and Community Psychiatry 44(2): 134–140

Gelder M, Mayou R, Geddes J 1999 Psychiatry, 2nd edn. Oxford University Press, Oxford

Ghaziuddin M 1998 Behavioural disorder in the mentally handicapped: the role of life events. British Journal of Psychiatry 152: 683–686

Ghaziuddin M, Alessi N, Greden J 1995 Life events and depression in children with pervasive developmental disorders. Journal of Autism and Developmental Disorders 25: 495–502

Ghaziuddin M, Ghaziuddin N, Greden J 2002 Depression in persons with autism: implications for research and clinical care. Journal of Autism and Developmental Disorders 32(4): 299–306

Goldstein G, Minshaw N J, Allen D N et al 2002 High-functioning autism and schizophrenia: a comparison of an early and late onset neurodevelopmental disorder. Archives of Clinical Neuropsychology 17: 461–475

Hall S 2001 Self-injurious behaviour in young children with Lesch–Nyhan syndrome. Developmental Medicine and Child Neurology 43: 745–749

Kanner L, Eisenberg L 1956 Early infantile autism 1943–1955. American Journal of Orthopsychiatry 26: 55–65

Konstantareas M M, Hewitt T 2001 Autistic disorder and schizophrenia: diagnostic overlaps. Journal of Autism and Developmental Disorders 31(1): 19–28

Le Couteur A L, Phillips W, Rutter M 1995 A broader phenotype of autism: the clinical spectrum in twins. Journal of Child Psychology and Psychiatry 37: 785–801

Lemma A 1996 Introduction to psychopathology. Sage, London

Mann A, Jenkins R, Cutting J et al 1981 The development of a standardized measure of abnormal personality. Psychological Medicine 11: 839–847

Matson J L, Mayville E A, Lott J D et al 2003 A comparison of social and adaptive functioning in persons with psychosis, autism and severe or profound mental retardation. Journal of Developmental and Physical Disabilities 15(1): 57–65

McBrien J 2003 The intellectually disordered offender: methodological problems in identification. Journal of Applied Research in Developmental Disabilities 16: 95–105

Mental Health Act 1983 HMSO, London

Mental Health Foundation 2000 The cost of autistic spectrum disorder. Updates 1(17)

Mullins J L, Christian L 2001 The effects of progressive relaxation training on the disruptive behavior of a boy with autism. Research in Developmental Disabilities 22: 449–462

Murphy G, Mason J 1999 People with developmental disabilities who offend. In: Bouras N (ed) Psychiatric and behavioural disorders in developmental disabilities and mental retardation. Cambridge University Press, Cambridge, p 226–246

Naik B I, Gangadharan S, Alexander R T 2002 Personality disorders in learning disability – the clinical experience. British Journal of Developmental Disabilities 48(2): 95–100

Nasr A, Roy M 2000 Association of a balanced chromosomal translocation (4;12)(q21.3;q15), affective disorder and autism. Journal of Intellectual Disability Research 44(2): 170–174

Reid A H, Ballinger B R 1987 Personality disorder in mental handicap. Psychological Medicine 17: 983–987

Rojahn J, Matson J L, Lott D et al 2002 The Behaviour Problems Inventory: an instrument for the assessment of self-injury, stereotypical behaviour and aggression/destructive behaviour in individuals with developmental disorders. Journal of Autism and Developmental Disorders 31: 577–588

Royal College of Psychiatrists 2001 DC-LD (Diagnostic criteria for psychiatric disorders for use with adults with learning disability/mental retardation). Occasional paper OP48. Gaskell, London

Shattock P 1997 The role of vaccines. Online. Available: www.osiris.sunderland.ac.uk/autism/vaccine.htm

Wing L 1981 Asperger's syndrome: a clinical account. Psychological Medicine 11: 115–119

World Health Organization 1992 ICD-10: The international statistical classification of diseases and related health problems, 10th revision. WHO, Geneva

Assessment tools

INTRODUCTION

Given the difficulties outlined in previous chapters of identifying and accurately describing the presence of mental health problems in people with learning disabilities, it is crucial that carers have access to, and training in, the use of appropriate, valid, and reliable assessment tools. Although the ultimate responsibility for diagnosing and treating mental health problems lies with the client's general practitioner or psychiatrist, the role of family members and carers in the initial identification and assessment of these problems cannot be overemphasised.

This chapter will, therefore, describe and evaluate a range of classification, diagnostic, screening, and assessment tools that may assist in the identification of mental health problems. The role of DSM-IV, ICD-10, and its learning disabilities version (DC-LD) in the assessment and diagnosis of mental health problems will be evaluated, with particular reference to the issue of labelling. Consideration will be given not only to those tools that are designed to be used within the general population but also to those that have been developed specifically for use with people with learning disabilities and with differing degrees of disability. These will include screening tools, psychiatric interview schedules, outcome measures, and behavioural assessment tools. This chapter will identify those tools that may be accessed and utilised by care workers, with a particular emphasis on tools that are readily available to practitioners within the UK. Most tools require some training in their use, and details of training requirements can normally be obtained from the tool developers. Contact details are provided in Appendix 2.

THE PURPOSE OF ASSESSMENT

In Chapters 2, 4 and 5, a range of explanations for the onset and existence of mental health problems in people with and without learning disabilities was explored. However, regardless of whichever model or explanation we adopt, it is necessary to identify and address the unique problems experienced by individuals in relation to their mental health needs. There are many reasons why we need to carry out a full and detailed assessment of the mental health needs of clients with learning disabilities. Primarily, we need to have a comprehensive overview of the client's current situation in order to provide a baseline against which to monitor changes over time. From this, we can then – in conjunction with the client, family and other carers – plan, implement, and evaluate interventions and care, predict future needs, and identify any risk factors. A thorough assessment can allow us to provide evidence and documentation to support our actions and decisions, and to communicate these to family members and carers. Finally, the information that we gather can assist the client's doctor in making a formal diagnosis which will allow for the prescription of appropriate treatment.

Formal diagnosis and labelling

In Chapters 3 and 4 we introduced some standard classification systems which can facilitate the arrival at a clear diagnosis and the prescription of appropriate treatment and care. We noted that standard classification systems can provide access to common definitions and terminology, and are central to communication between professionals locally, nationally, and internationally.

However, while arrival at a formal diagnosis is important, it is not without its difficulties. One of the key disadvantages of having such classification and diagnostic systems is that they equip clients with a 'label' that often becomes difficult to lose or change, and which might increase the social stigma and exclusion already often experienced by people with learning disabilities. Furthermore, classification systems can create boundaries between professionals, carers, and clients, in that professionals can use technical language and jargon to the exclusion of clients and carers, thus creating communication barriers.

It could be argued, though, that the advantages that come with diagnoses and labels can outweigh these disadvantages. Labels can facilitate access to a range of relevant services, skills, and knowledge, as well as ending the often long and painful search to identify the precise nature of a client's problems. With this debate in mind, we present below a review of the development of classification systems and diagnostic tools that may enhance the identification of mental health problems in people with learning disabilities.

MENTAL HEALTH CLASSIFICATION SYSTEMS

To assist in the process of assessment and diagnosis, there exists a range of classification systems and diagnostic tools that aim to provide a common language and shared understanding between health care professionals, and we have referred to some of these in previous chapters of the book. How did these tools originate? In the early 20th century it was noticed that symptoms of mental health problems tended to occur together, and consequently the first system of classification of mental disorder was developed.

Building on this early work, in 1952 the *Diagnostic and Statistical Manual* was first introduced by the American Psychiatric Association. It has undergone many revisions, the latest version being DSM-IV-TR (American Psychiatric Association 2000). This manual, the key reference in use in America and also widely consulted in its international version in the UK, aims to provide a comprehensive classification of mental health problems. It lists around 300 disorders defined in terms of observable symptoms that psychiatrists can use to make a formal diagnosis of mental health problems.

Similarly, the ICD-10, the tenth version of the *International Classification of Diseases* (World Health Organization 1992), provides a list of symptoms and diagnostic criteria, and is popular throughout Europe. Both tools specify how many symptoms, experienced over what period of time, are necessary for the psychiatrist to make a diagnosis. For example, using ICD-10, a psychiatrist might make a diagnosis of schizophrenia if one out of a list of eight primary symptoms has been present for at least a month. Using DSM-IV, the same psychiatrist would need to identify the presence of two or more from a list of five primary symptoms occurring over a 1-month period. However, DSM-IV requires, in addition, that signs of disturbance have been persistent for at least 6 months before a diagnosis is made.

Classification systems and people with learning disabilities

It is important to have a reliable and valid classification system with which to assess and diagnose mental health problems in people with learning disabilities, in order that they can access appropriate interventions and services (Charlot 2003). Until recently, however, a psychiatrist attempting to diagnose the presence of a mental health problem in someone with learning disabilities would have had to rely on a tool developed for the general population. However, it has been shown that neither DSM-IV nor ICD-10 is fully compatible when making a psychiatric diagnosis in people with learning disabilities (Deb et al 2001). Clarke et al (1994), for example, used the ICD-10 to categorise psychiatric and behavioural abnormalities among people with learning disabilities, made recommendations for changes to some diagnostic criteria and the methods of coding diagnoses, and stressed the need for additional guidelines when classifying disorders associated with mental retardation. Einfeld & Tonge (1999) concluded that there were some areas of uncertainty even when using the ICD-10 guide for mental retardation (World Health Organization 1996), for example when attempting to assess for Asperger syndrome.

In response to such observed deficiencies, the Royal College of Psychiatrists introduced the DC-LD (Diagnostic criteria for psychiatric disorders for use with adults with learning disabilities/mental retardation) in 2001. The authors wanted to improve upon existing classification tools designed for the general population and to make them more appropriate for the learning disabled population. DC-LD can be used by psychiatrists as a 'stand-alone' tool for people with moderate to profound learning disabilities, but it should be used, if necessary, in conjunction with ICD-10 for people with mild learning disabilities. Cross-references to DSM-IV codes are made within DC-LD, making it perhaps the most comprehensive and useful tool for practitioners in this field in the UK.

At around the same time, the European Association for Mental Health in Mental Retardation (EAMHMR) produced the first in a series of practice guidelines designed to promote evidence based practice, and to describe symptoms associated with different psychiatric illnesses for use as a reference point for all professionals and carers working with adults with learning disabilities (Deb et al 2001). In this way, the book aimed to raise awareness of mental health problems and to promote appropriate referral for people with learning disabilities.

Although the three classification tools/diagnostic guides described above are primarily intended for use by psychiatrists, there is no doubt that direct care staff can support and inform medical practitioners in making their diagnosis by providing accurate assessment information. In addition to using the tools to assist with diagnosis, a psychiatrist will normally take a full and detailed history in a systematic way, and carers will contribute extensively to the gathering of these data. Deb et al (2001) recommend a set of components for comprehensive history taking for people with learning disabilities, and these are summarised in Box 6.1.

In some cases, of course, it will not be possible to elicit some or all of this information from the client. In these cases it will be necessary to ask another person, such as the main carer, to describe the current problem and any relevant history. To this end, carers will need to draw upon a wide range of assessment methods and skills to provide as comprehensive data as possible. These assessment methods are described below.

Box 6.1   Components of a comprehensive history

- Family history
- Personal and development history – including relationships and important life events
- Medical history – including physical illness and disability
- Psychiatric history – including previous contact with mental health services
- Social history – including employment, housing, and levels of social support
- Drug history – including past and present medication and its effects, plus any substance or alcohol use, if relevant
- Forensic history, i.e. problems with the law, if relevant
- History of the presenting complaint

For more detail, see Deb et al (2001).

ASSESSMENT METHODS

We have at our disposal a wide range of ways of gathering information about our clients, and in particular of picking up clues that they might be experiencing some mental health problems. As we saw in Chapter 3, ratings by a significant other, clinical interviews, and self-reporting by the client are key methods for obtaining assessment data, but observation is also a significant tool. Some methods are used in everyday work and interactions with clients; others are more formal. These might include, for example, a continuous period of *direct observation*, or carrying out a detailed observation at set intervals of time. *Interviews*, either with clients themselves or with someone who has a detailed knowledge of them, may be unstructured, with the interviewer deciding on what questions to ask as the interview progresses, or they may be highly structured, such that the interviewer has to ask a set list of questions in a predetermined order. Finally, we may draw upon *standardised assessment tools* such as questionnaires and rating scales. It is important that the outcomes of assessment are recorded in order that changes over time can be tracked and adjustments to intervention strategies made. All of these assessment methods require knowledge and skill on the part of the carer, and have implications for the ongoing education and training of care staff.

A range of standardised assessment tools is described later in this chapter, but one problem that faces us is which tool to choose, and how to ensure that it will help in identifying the unique needs of our clients.

What makes a good assessment tool?

According to Tunmore (2000), a good assessment tool will have been piloted – that is, tried out on a sample of people who are similar to those for whom the tool is intended – to ensure that the language and terminology used within it are clear, and that there is no ambiguity in meaning. The tool should also be easy to use, with a clear scoring system and explanation of the results of the scores obtained. The timescale for completion of the tool should not be so long that the assessor and the client become tired or bored. Most tools require at least some training in their use, but this should not take so long or be so expensive that care staff will be unwilling or unable to access it. Finally, a good tool must be both valid and reliable.

Validity

In order for a tool to be valid, it must assess what the user wishes to assess. It should cover all relevant aspects of the topic and compare well with other tools and other ways of collecting information. In order to be valid, a tool must also be reliable.

Reliability

This means that the tool should provide the same sort of information each time it is used, and furthermore, two or more different assessors using the same tool should produce the same results.

Enhancing validity and reliability

In order to enhance validity and reliability, it is possible and desirable to collect data using more than one assessment method or tool. For example, the use of both observation *and* a rating scale would provide more information than one method alone, and in practice, when making an assessment, carers and others will normally take into account a wide range of sources of information, such as past records, history, interviews, observations, and formal tools.

Mental health screening tools for people with learning disabilities

The following section describes a range of informant-based tools (completed by carers on behalf of the client) that aim to screen for the presence of mental health problems in people with learning disabilities. However, it should be noted that not all tools in use have been tested for validity and reliability amongst people with learning disabilities, and information provided by carers on behalf of clients can be of questionable validity and reliability (Deb et al 2001, Kellet et al 2003, Ross & Oliver 2003). A screening tool does not necessarily provide a definitive diagnosis, rather it might prompt continued monitoring or referral for further investigation in specific areas of mental health functioning. There is an apparent under-representation of tests designed solely for people with severe and profound learning disabilities (Ross & Oliver 2003, Sturmey et al 1991); however the DASH-II (Matson 1995) is designed specifically for this client group.

Assessment of Dual Diagnosis (ADD) (Matson & Bamburg 1998)

This is a 79-item American-designed screening instrument for people with mild or moderate learning disabilities. It has 13 subscales (mania, depression, anxiety, post-traumatic stress disorder, substance abuse, somatoform disorder, dementia, conduct disorder, pervasive developmental disorder, schizophrenia, personality disorder, eating disorder, and sexual disorder) which assess the frequency, duration, and severity of symptoms, particularly those occurring within the preceding month. The ADD is related to DSM-IV (American Psychiatric Association 1994), and has been tested for reliability by the developers. It can be used by health care professionals with training, and takes approximately 20 minutes to complete. Although threshold scores are not provided (scores beyond which are indicative of a problem), the test developers suggest that once the assessor has established which problems are occurring most frequently, then duration and severity can be examined to see whether a diagnosis can be warranted.

Diagnostic Assessment for the Severely Handicapped-II (DASH-II) (Matson 1995)

This is an American-designed tool comprising 84 items representing 13 diagnostic categories (anxiety, depression, mania, pervasive developmental disorder/autism, schizophrenia, stereotyped behaviour, self-injurious behaviour, elimination disorders, eating disorders, sleep disorders, sexual disorders, organic syndromes, and impulse control). It has a similar format to ADD, but is designed specifically for people with severe and profound disabilities. Problems are rated for frequency, duration, and severity. The DASH-II takes between 20 and 30 minutes to complete and should be administered by a health or social care professional who interviews a carer who has known the client for at least 6 months. Threshold scores are provided for eight of the diagnostic categories; scores beyond these call for further assessment in the relevant problem area.

PAS-ADD instruments

The Psychiatric Assessment Schedule for Adults with Developmental Disabilities (PAS-ADD) is a British-designed tool that offers a multi-level approach to the identification and assessment of mental health problems in people with learning disabilities. The first two levels, namely the PAS-ADD Checklist and the Mini PAS-ADD, are informant-rated screening tools while the third, the PAS-ADD Interview, allows for a more detailed assessment to be made by a trained professional. The PAS-ADD Interview is described later in this chapter.

PAS-ADD Checklist (Moss et al 1998). This is a screening tool designed specifically for use by direct care staff or family members, to assist them in recognising mental health problems in their clients, and to facilitate referral to an appropriate professional if required. The tool comprises a checklist of life events that have happened in the past year and takes approximately 15 minutes to complete. Twenty-nine symptom items in seven broad areas are scored according to whether they have been a serious problem or a problem for the person in the past 4 weeks; have happened but have not been a problem; or have not happened. These broad areas are appetite and sleep, tension and worry, phobias and panics, depression and hypomania, obsessions and compulsions, psychoses, and autism. Threshold scores are provided for each of the seven areas, and clients scoring above the threshold could be considered to be at risk. The checklist has been found to have acceptable levels of validity and reliability (Moss et al 1998).

Mini PAS-ADD (Prosser et al 1996). The Mini PAS-ADD is an assessment schedule that can be used when the PAS-ADD Checklist has identified a possible area of risk. Taking approximately 30–40 minutes to administer, the Checklist should be completed by a carer who has known the client for at least 6 months. It asks questions about life events that might be triggers to or causes of current difficulties, plus 86 items based on the client's health and behaviour over the past 4 weeks, to be rated as mild (score = 0), moderate (score = 1), or severe (score = 2). After rating, problem areas are identified on seven scales: depression, anxiety, hypomania/mania, obsessive–compulsive, psychosis, unspecified disorders, and developmental disorders. A threshold score is provided for each scale, and scores equal to or above the threshold in one or more of the scales suggest that a referral for further psychiatric investigation should be made. Validity and reliability have been demonstrated (Prosser et al 1998).

Reiss Screen for Maladaptive Behaviour (Reiss 1994)

This screening tool is designed for those aged over 12 with learning disabilities. It aims to facilitate the identification of mental health problems in people with learning disabilities, in order to assist them to receive the appropriate mental health services and interventions. The screening tool measures the likelihood that a client has a significant mental health problem, and it claims to be useful with mild, moderate, and severe degrees of learning disabilities. It is completed by care workers who have known the client reasonably well for at least 3 months prior to testing. Two or more raters are recommended, which will enhance the reliability of the screening.

The test takes about 20 minutes to complete, and includes 38 items covering eight scales (aggressive behaviour, psychosis, paranoia, depression [behavioural and physical signs], dependent personality disorder, avoidant disorder, and autism). Raters judge each item as currently no problem (score = 0), a problem (score = 1), or a major problem (score = 2). The mean average from the scores of the two raters is calculated. In addition, the mean scores of 26 of the 38 items are totalled to arrive at an overall severity score. Computer software is available to assist with analysis, or tests can be posted to the test developers for analysis. Otherwise, the person carrying out the test can score it manually, and by comparing scores in the eight areas against norm scores, the tester can identify specific problem areas and the severity of problems in that area. In other words, if any score is above a suggested cut-off point, then the client should be referred to a mental health professional for further investigations. This tool has been subjected to numerous assessments of validity and reliability.

Interview schedules

While screening tools are extremely useful in gaining some insight into the type and severity of problems experienced by clients, and to prompt for a referral to an appropriate professional if necessary, they cannot provide in-depth information. Where this is required, more extensive data can be gathered through interviewing clients and carers. Furthermore, informant-based tools cannot access the client's unique experiences directly. Clinical interviewing, on the other hand, enables access to the individual's first-hand experience of mental health problems and symptoms. However, being able to interview people with a mental health problem, particularly when coupled with learning disabilities, presents some major obstacles and requires a high level of expertise (Moss et al 1993). Hence, some interview schedules are designed primarily for use by appropriately trained medical staff. Others, however, such as the KGV scale, may be used by professional care workers, given appropriate training. Deb et al (2001) and Prosser & Bromley (1998) provide useful guidelines for interviewing people with learning disabilities who may have mental health problems, and these are summarised below.

Interviewing people with learning disabilities

Wherever possible, the interview should take place in a setting familiar to the client, ideally one that the client chooses. The interviewer should know the client prior to the interview taking place, but this is not always possible, particularly when the client has been referred to a specialist for the first time. Other people attending the interview such as carers and family members should have a good relationship with the client, but should not offer information unless it is specifically requested, allowing the client, where possible, to answer questions personally. The client should, if possible, consent to other people being present at the interview. There should be flexibility in relation to the length of interview. For example, it should be possible to split the interview into several shorter sessions if the client is likely to get tired or bored, or lose concentration.

The interviewer should prepare well for the interview. Knowledge of the client's communication and linguistic ability will allow for the prior preparation of appropriate visual aids such as pictures to support the topic areas to be covered in the interview, and for consideration of appropriate language to be used in the interview. The interview should be opened with an explanation of its purpose, and its expected duration, and issues of consent and confidentiality should be clarified at the outset.

During the interview, questions should be as short and simple as possible, and the interviewer should not confuse the client by asking two questions in one. Neither should leading questions such as 'You're happy here, aren't you?' be used. Questions should be sufficiently open to allow the client to answer in his or her own way, but the interviewer should be prepared to reword or follow up questions to elicit more precise answers, obtain examples, or clarify issues as necessary. An example of an open question might be 'Can you tell me how you are feeling at the moment', and a follow-up question to the response 'I feel sad' might be 'Can you tell me more about feeling sad?'. Closed questions can be useful to obtain precise information, particularly if they take the form of 'either-or'. When interviewing carers to gain additional information, the same general principles apply.

A range of assessment tools that require interviewing skills are outlined below. The CAN and the KGV scale are not designed specifically for people with learning disabilities but may be useful for those with mild levels of disability and good communication skills.

CAN (Camberwell Assessment of Need) (Slade et al 1999)

This is a British tool designed for people with a severe mental illness that was originally intended to assist local authorities in assessing patients' needs for community services. It aims to identify social as well as clinical needs as a basis for planning appropriate care. The tool takes around 25 minutes to complete, and rates 22 areas of need as 'no serious problem', 'moderate problem', or 'current serious problem'. It then asks about the level of help needed and received for each problem. The tool is judged to be both valid and reliable by its developers. Subsequently, a range of versions of CAN have been developed for specific populations, one of which is CANDID, designed for people with learning disabilities who may have mental health problems, and this is described below.

CANDID (Camberwell Assessment of Need for Adults with Developmental and Intellectual Disabilities) (Xenitidis et al 2000)

This is a version of the Camberwell Assessment of Need (CAN) tool. The CANDID maintains the same format and structure as the CAN, but has been modified to make its content relevant to adults with learning disabilities and mental health problems. CANDID aims to record separately the views of clients and formal and informal carers via semi-structured interviews (any or all three may be interviewed in parallel). The 25 broad areas of need, including mental health need, are rated according to 'no serious need', 'met need', 'unmet need', or 'not known'.

There are two versions, CANDID-R, for research use, and CANDID-S, a short version for clinical and research purposes. A range of care workers can complete CANDID, and formal training is not a requirement, although the interviewer needs to have experience of clinical assessment. CANDID-R takes 20–30 minutes to complete, whereas CANDID-S takes 10–15 minutes.

The tools are claimed to be valid and reliable, and have been found to be acceptable for community and hospital settings (Xenitidis et al 2000). When aggregated, results can inform resource allocation and service planning.

PAS-ADD Interview (Moss et al 1996a)

This is a semi-structured clinical interview based on ICD-10 (World Health Organization 1992), conducted once with the client and once with a key informant, either of which can detect symptoms and produce diagnoses. It takes upwards of 30 minutes to conduct, depending on the range and severity of mental health problems. It uses a computer algorithm to produce diagnoses and other diagnostic information in conjunction with ICD-10 (World Health Organization 1992). The interview has good reliability when compared with the clinical opinion of psychiatrists (Moss et al 1997).

KGV (Manchester) Scale (Krawiecka et al 1977)

This is a 14-item interview schedule designed for assessing symptoms and experiences of mental health problems (particularly psychosis) in the general population, and to enable regular and accurate monitoring. It combines the patient's self-report with the rater's observations of physical and non-verbal signs, and – by providing a range of mandatory questions and examples of supplementary questions should the patient's answers to the mandatory questions be inadequate – it relies on skilled interviewing technique. It is suitable for use with people with mild learning disabilities, and forms part of the LDCNS tool (see below).

The Learning Disabilities Version of the Cardinal Needs Schedule (LDCNS) (Raghavan et al 2001)

This has been adapted for people with learning disabilities from the Cardinal Needs Schedule (Marshall et al 1995). It offers a systematic and comprehensive battery of measures and instruments including interviews and rating scales. Interviews (with clients and carers) are designed with a high degree of structure and cover a wide range of areas that extends beyond mental health issues. The schedule incorporates the revised Manchester (KGV) scale (Krawiecka et al 1977) and other standardised scales. Supplementary questions can be used to identify dementia or dangerousness, and auxiliary schedules may be used if appropriate to screen for substance misuse. Responses can be entered directly into the computer program 'Autoneed' (Lockwood 2001) for scoring. The aim is to identify which of the problems identified are *cardinal*, in other words, severe enough or stressful enough to require action.

This schedule differs from others in that, having identified whether problems are cardinal, a list of suitable interventions that have not previously been offered to the client is suggested (Raghavan 2000). The tool may be used by professionals including psychiatrists, psychologists, occupational therapists, social workers, nurses, and other support professionals, and workplace based training is required to carry out the data input and needs analysis.

Outcome measures

Outcome measures aim to assess the effects of intervention. A baseline measure is obtained prior to intervention, and subsequent measures are obtained regularly following intervention to evaluate the success or otherwise of interventions in a range of areas. Interventions can then be adjusted or removed, or new interventions added, according to these outcomes.

Brief Symptom Inventory (BSI) (Derogatis 1993)

This is a shortened version of the Symptom Checklist 90-R (SCL-90-R) (Derogatis 1983), a widely used tool for measuring the effectiveness of psychotherapy, and which has also been used with people with learning disabilities. The BSI is a 53-item self-report inventory scored on a 5-point scale, which identifies nine primary symptom dimensions (somatisation, obsessive–compulsive, interpersonal sensitivity, depression, anxiety, hostility, phobic anxiety, paranoid ideation, and psychoticism). It has been used successfully as an outcome measure in mental health intervention studies, and may be a more appropriate outcome measure for people with learning disabilities than SCL-90-R as it is relatively short. Kellet et al (2003) have shown that the BSI is a reasonably reliable tool, applicable in a range of settings, and which should be considered as a useful tool to examine the effectiveness of a wide range of clinical interventions in people with learning disabilities.

Health of the Nation Outcome Scales (HoNOS) (Wing et al 1996)

In response to the *Health of the Nation* strategy (Department of Health 1992) these scales have been developed and validated for use with people with mental health problems in the general population, with the aim of improving the health and social functioning of mentally ill people. The scales provide a numerical record that draws on a wide range of information. They are designed for use by professionals and provide a systematic summary of behaviours and functioning, which can serve as a baseline against which future outcomes can be measured. Twelve items are graded for severity on a 5-point scale, and there is a framework to measure risk and vulnerability.

These scales have been shown to be a useful global measure of mental health status. Subsequent versions include a HoNOS scale for people with learning disabilities, which is described below.

The Health of the Nation Outcome Scales for people with learning disabilities (HoNOS-LD) (Roy et al 2002)

These are HoNOS scales recalibrated to suit the needs of people with learning disabilities. They are suitable for all degrees of disability, and provide an easy-to-use instrument that can measure change or lack of change in the level of functioning of people with learning disabilities who also have mental health needs. The informant needs to know the client well, but the scales specifically measure changes within a 4 week period. The 18 items are rated on a scale of 0 = 'no problem during period rated', 1 = 'mild problem', 2 = 'moderate problem', 3 = 'severe problem', 4 = 'very severe problem'. There is good inter-rater validity and reliability, and the scale correlates well with the Aberrant Behaviour Checklist (see below). Although designed for use by mental health professionals with appropriate training, the outcomes identified can be used by carers in planning interventions. The scales can be analysed using accompanying computer software.

TOOLS FOR THE ASSESSMENT OF SPECIFIC DEFICITS OR DISORDERS

All the tools described so far screen or test for a wide range of mental health problems. However, in some cases, where a specific problem is suspected, it may be more useful to select a specific tool to assess for the presence or severity of that problem. There are countless such tools available, but very few that are specifically designed for people with learning disabilities. However, some of these may be suitable for people with mild or moderate levels of learning disability, or have been adapted for that purpose. A selection of specific tools is presented below.

Tools for mood (affective) disorders

As noted in Chapter 4, Marston et al (1997) suggested that a specific assessment tool may be needed to identify behavioural depressive equivalents such as screaming, self-injurious behaviour, reduced communication, and social isolation in people with severe or profound levels of disability, and have designed an informant checklist of 30 depression items suitable for all levels of disability. Others have argued that existing tools may be adequate for the assessment of depression, but Ross & Oliver (2003) point out that many of these are not suitable for people with severe and profound learning disabilities, and further research and testing is required. A selection of tools that might be suitable for people with mild or moderate levels of learning disabilities is presented below.

The *Beck Depression Inventory* (BDI) (Beck et al 1996) is a 21-item self-rating tool containing item statements such as 'I have lost interest in other people', to be rated on a 4-point scale, ranging from 0 to 3. Test scores of 11 or more indicate some mood disturbance; scores of over 25 indicate clinical depression. Beck et al (1974) have also designed a brief scale to measure the risk of suicide, known as the *Hopelessness Scale*.

Other tools which have been used effectively with people with learning disabilities (Sturmey et al 1991) are the *Hamilton Rating Scale for Depression* (Hamilton 1967), an 18-item scale which can be completed during an interview, but which may have some structural weaknesses (Barker 1997), and the *Zung Self-rating Depression Scale* (Zung 1965). This comprises 20 items to be rated on a 4-point scale (none or a little of the time, some of the time, a good part of the time, most or all of the time).

Both the BDI and the Zung scale are reported as being successful for people with learning disabilities and depression (Lindsay 1999, Powell 2003), and item statements may be read out to those clients who are unable to read.

Tools for neurotic and stress-related disorders

- The *Hamilton Anxiety Scale* (Hamilton 1959) has a similar structure to the Hamilton Depression Scale, consisting of 14 items defined by a series of symptoms rated on a 5-point scale (0 = not present to 4 = severe).
- The *Hospital Anxiety and Depression (HAD) Scale* (Zigmond & Snaith 1983) is, as the title suggests, a brief assessment of anxiety and depression, consisting of 14 items divided into two subscales. Designed for use in the general population, it is nonetheless written in an easy-to-understand language that might make it suitable for people with learning disabilities. Items to be rated include: 'I feel tense and wound up' and 'I have lost interest in my appearance'. Respondents rate their answers on a 4-point scale with the total scores for each subscale ranging from 0 to 21. A score of 11 or above is considered clinically significant.
- The *Zung Self-rating Anxiety Scale* (Zung 1971) has a similar format to the Zung Depression Scale, and comprises 20 items to be rated on a 4-point scale (none or a little of the time, some of the time, a good part

of the time, most or all of the time). This is one of the standard anxiety assessment tools, but as people with learning disabilities may find it difficult to objectively rate themselves, it has been adapted for people with learning disabilities by Lindsay & Michie (1988). Items are read out to clients and can be reworded if not understood. Supplementary questions are provided.

- The *Compulsive Behaviour Checklist* (Gedye 1992) is devised specifically for people with learning disabilities, and is completed by carers.

Tools for psychotic disorders/schizophrenia

Psychiatrists will typically call upon standardised diagnostic criteria when interviewing clients to diagnose schizophrenia. Although there has been little research in relation to the development of an appropriate measure of schizophrenia for people with learning disabilities (Sturmey et al 1991), many of the tools already described are suitable for care staff use. Meadows et al (1991) demonstrated that as symptoms of schizophrenia are broadly similar in people with learning disabilities and those without, then a standardised diagnostic interview such as would be used within the general population was acceptable for people with learning disabilities. The KGV scale (incorporated within LDCNS, Raghavan et al 2001) offers a structured approach to the identification of delusions, hallucinations, thought disorder, and negative symptoms of schizophrenia, through interview and observations, and the schizophrenia section of the PAS-ADD instruments goes some way towards the effective identification of schizophrenia (Moss et al 1996b). Until specific tools are developed to assess for the presence of symptoms of schizophrenia in people with learning disabilities, either general population tools or broad based mental health assessment tools can be used effectively.

Tools for organic disorders/dementias

As with other problems, cognitive deterioration and dementia are difficult to assess in people with learning disabilities, particularly since memory and orientation impairments are difficult to observe directly (Evenhuis 1992). A range of tools that may contribute to the assessment and diagnosis process is outlined below.

Mini-Mental State Examination (MMSE) (Folstein et al 1975)

This is a brief, quantitative screening tool for cognitive state, i.e., it tests short-term memory, attention, orientation, language, and ability to calculate. It is frequently used in the UK to assess cognitive deterioration and possible dementia in older people. A test score of 30 is possible; it is suggested that additional testing is carried out for clients who score less than 26, and the test should be repeated at intervals to identify change over time. Although it is not designed specifically for people with learning disabilities, it is suitable for those with mild learning disabilities, provided that they do not have reading or writing difficulties (Sturmey et al 1991), and may be useful for detecting the onset of dementia, particularly in people with Down's syndrome.

Dementia Questionnaire for Persons with Mental Retardation (DMR) (Evenhuis et al 1990)

This screening tool is designed to be completed by a carer on behalf of the client, taking the past 2 months' behaviour into account. It measures cognitive and social skills via 50 questions in eight categories: short-term memory, long-term memory, spatial and temporal orientation, speech, practical skills, mood, activity and interest, and behavioural disturbance. Responses can be 0 = normally yes; 1 = sometimes; 2 = normally no. Cognitive and social scores can be calculated separately.

Ideally the test should be repeated over a period of several years to note changes indicative of dementia. Although the developers claim the tool is suitable for people with Down's syndrome, Prasher (1997) has suggested some changes to the scoring criteria to make it suitable for this population.

Dementia scale for Down syndrome (Gedye 1995)

This is a more specific tool for people with Down's syndrome, through which two informants are interviewed about changes in the client's cognitive and daily living skills. It is possible, using this tool, to identify stage of dementia as early, middle or late, and also to differentiate Alzheimer's disease from depression and other physical problems.

Burt & Aylward (2000) in the USA have suggested that a test battery be completed to diagnose dementia in people with learning disabilities. This includes the DMR, Gedye scale, and Reiss screen, together with tests to measure stress, memory, and the ability to carry out simple commands. However, while carers would be crucial in the administration, the decision to implement such a battery of tests would lie with the client's psychiatrist.

Behavioural assessment tools

For many years, tools have been available to assess behavioural difficulties in people with learning disabilities. As we noted in Chapter 3, it is often difficult to distinguish between challenging behaviours and mental health problems in people with learning disabilities, so in these cases it may be useful to include behavioural assessment tools as part of the overall strategy to try to identify the precise nature of the problems experienced by the client. Three such tools are evaluated below.

Aberrant Behaviour Checklist (ABC) (Aman et al 1985)

Developed in the mid 1980s, this tool is designed to measure the effects of treatment and to assess general behaviour problems in people with learning disabilities. It was originally designed for people in residential services but it can also be used with people living in the community, and for children as well as adults (Aman et al 1995). It can be used for people with moderate to severe levels of learning disabilities, and measures five factors: irritability, lethargy, stereotypy, hyperactivity, and inappropriate speech.

Although this tool is sometimes used as an instrument to detect psychopathology in people with learning disabilities, it is not recommended solely for this purpose as it is designed to measure behaviour problems and not mental disorders (Reiss & Valenti-Hein 1994). However, it may be a useful supplement to other assessment strategies such as the DASH-II, particularly for people with severe and profound levels of learning disability (Paclawskyj et al 1997).

Functional Analysis of Problem Behaviour (O'Neill et al 1997)

Functional behavioural analysis, as assessed via this tool, is a systematic approach to understanding the relationship between behaviour and aspects of the environment that predict and maintain it. Functional analysis normally includes a review of the client's records, direct observations of behaviour, and interviews.

Motivation Assessment Scale (MAS) (Durand & Crimmins 1988)

This is a 16-item questionnaire completed by care staff that helps to assess the functional significance of behaviour, based on the notion that all behaviour has a function for the individual. It aims to identify the specific effects of particular behaviours for the individual, such as gaining social attention or escaping from perceived demands.

Exercise

Reflect back on the stories of Geoff, Jason, Jenny, and David who have been introduced in the book so far. In each case, consider which, if any, of the assessment tools outlined in the chapter might be useful in trying to gain a clear understanding of their problems. Give reasons for your choices in each case.

All of our clients will benefit from a thorough physical examination to exclude any physiological cause for their current experiences. Following this, a screening tool such as the Mini PAS-ADD in each case will help to identify the broad areas in which they might be experiencing most difficulty.

Any score above the given threshold would give an indication as to which problem areas should be explored further.

Jason has good cognitive and linguistic abilities and will be able to give an account of his experiences directly, once his cooperation and trust have been obtained, hence a self-report tool or structured interview would be useful. Geoff, Jenny, and David have more limited intellectual abilities, and may be less able to communicate their experiences directly, but all efforts to obtain their views must be made with the use of appropriate visual aids such as cue cards or photographs (e.g. Holland et al 1998).

Jenny has severe learning disabilities, so it might be helpful for her carers to complete either the Reiss screen or the DASH-II on her behalf. Jeff is expressing verbal aggression and shouting. Could these be expressions of depression? If we think this might be the case, he might benefit from screening specifically for depression.

Both David and Jenny display self-injurious behaviour. As we saw in Chapter 5, several causes of learning disabilities have self-injurious behaviour as a feature, hence one of the behavioural assessment tools might be useful, but we should not assume that this is a manifestation of the learning disability, and should aim to uncover their feelings using appropriate tools. However, just as a spade is merely a tool to aid the task of digging the garden, so too are assessment tools merely aids to the task of comprehensive mental health assessment. Whichever tools are chosen, they should be treated precisely as aids, as they are no substitute for skilful observation, careful communication, and accurate recording on the part of the carer.

CONCLUSION

This chapter has presented a range of diagnostic and assessment tools that might assist in the process of identifying mental health problems in people with learning disabilities, both in terms of the type of problem and its severity. Screening tools are particularly useful in identifying areas in which there might be problems, and in providing supportive evidence for further assessment or referral to specialist services. However, it should be noted that no tool is perfect, and although it can provide valuable information, it is no substitute for thorough observations and reporting of clients' mood and behaviour by direct care staff. Neither can any single tool be relied upon to provide all the data required to assess/diagnose a client as having a mental health problem. In order to provide as broad a picture as possible, a range of data sources and data collection methods should be used, in conjunction with a selection of relevant tools.

In Chapter 7, we explore a range of therapeutic interventions that can be considered once assessment has pointed the way to the key problem areas of the client.

REFERENCES

Aman M, Singh N, Stewart A 1985 The Aberrant Behaviour Checklist: a behaviour rating scale for the assessment of treatment effects. American Journal of Mental Deficiency 89: 485–491

Aman M, Burrow W, Wolford P 1995 The Aberrant Behaviour Checklist – Community: factor validity and effect of subject variables for adults in group homes. American Journal on Mental Retardation 100(3): 283–292

American Psychiatric Association 1994 Diagnostic and statistical manual of mental disorders DSM-IV, 4th edn. American Psychiatric Association, Washington

American Psychiatric Association 2000 Diagnostic and statistical manual of mental disorders DSM-IV-TR (Text Revision). American Psychiatric Association, Washington

Barker P 1997 Assessment in psychiatric and mental health nursing. Nelson Thornes, Cheltenham

Beck A, Weissman A, Lester D et al 1974 The measurement of pessimism: the hopelessness scale. Journal of Consulting and Clinical Psychology 42: 861–865

Beck A, Steer R, Brown G 1996 The Beck Depression Inventory II. Harcourt Brace & Co, San Antonio

Burt D B, Aylward E H 2000 Test battery for the diagnosis of dementia in individuals with intellectual disability. Journal of Intellectual Disability Research 44(2): 175–180

Charlot L 2003 Mission impossible? Developing an accurate classification of psychiatric disorders for individuals with developmental disabilities. Mental Health Aspects of Developmental Disabilities 6(1): 26–34

Clarke D J, Cumella S, Corbett J 1994 Use of ICD-10: research on diagnostic criteria to categorise psychiatric and behavioural abnormalities among people with learning disabilities. The West Midlands field trial. Mental Handicap Research 7(4): 273–284

Deb S, Matthews T, Holt G et al 2001 Practice guidelines for the assessment and diagnosis of mental health problems in adults with intellectual disability. Pavilion, Brighton

Department of Health 1992 Health of the nation. HMSO, London

Derogatis L 1983 SCL-90-R: administration, scoring and procedures: Manual II. Clinical Psychometric Research, Towson, MD

Derogatis L 1993 Brief Symptom Inventory: administration, scoring and procedures: Manual, 3rd edn. National Computer Systems, Minneapolis

Durand M, Crimmins D 1988 The MAS administration guide. Monaco, Topeka, KS

Einfeld S L, Tonge B J 1999 Observations on the use of the ICD-10 guide for mental retardation. Journal of Intellectual Disability Research 43(5): 408–412

Evenhuis H M 1992 Evaluation of a screening instrument for dementia in ageing mentally retarded persons. Journal of Intellectual Disability Research 36: 337–347

Evenhuis H, Kengen M, Eurlings H 1990 Dementia questionnaire for mentally retarded persons. Hooge Burch, PO Box 2027, 2470 AA Zwammerdam, The Netherlands

Folstein M, Folstein S, McHugh P 1975 'Mini-Mental State'. A practical method for grading the cognitive state of patients for the clinician. Journal of Psychiatric Research 12: 189–198

Gedye A 1992 Recognising obsessive–compulsive disorder claims in clients with developmental disabilities. The Habilitative Mental Health Care Newsletter 11: 73–74

Gedye A 1995 Dementia scale for Down syndrome. Gedye Research and Consulting, PO Box 39081, Vancouver, Canada

Hamilton M 1959 Hamilton anxiety scale. In: Schutte N, Malouff J 1995 Sourcebook of adult assessment strategies. Plenum Press, New York

Hamilton M 1967 Development of a rating scale for primary depressive illness. British Journal of Social and Clinical Psychology 6: 278–296

Holland A, Payne A, Vickey L 1998 Exploring your emotions (photographs and manual). BILD Publications, Plymouth

Kellett S, Beail N, Newman D et al 2003 Utility of the Brief Symptom Inventory in the assessment of psychological distress. Journal of Applied Research in Intellectual Disabilities 16: 127–134

Krawiecka M, Goldberg D, Vaughan M 1977 A standardised psychiatric assessment scale for rating chronic psychotic patients. Acta Psychiatrica Scandinavica 55: 299–308

Lindsay W R 1999 Cognitive therapy. The Psychologist 12: 238–241

Lindsay W R, Michie A M 1988 Adaptation of the Zung self-rating anxiety scale for people with a mental handicap. Journal of Mental Deficiency Research 32: 485–490

Lockwood A 2001 Autoneed (computerised version of the Cardinal Needs Schedule). www.gac.man.ac.uk/autoneed

Marshall M, Hogg L, Gath D et al 1995 Cardinal needs schedule: a modified version of the MRC Needs for Care Assessment Schedule. Psychological Medicine 25: 605–617

Marston G, Perry D, Roy A 1997 Manifestations of depression in people with intellectual disability. Journal of Intellectual Disability Research 41(6): 476–480

Matson J L 1995 The diagnostic assessment for the severely handicapped II. Scientific Publishers, Baton Rouge

Matson J L, Bamburg J W 1998 Reliability of the Assessment of Dual Diagnosis (ADD). Research in Developmental Disabilities 19(1): 89–95

Meadows G, Turner T, Campbell L et al 1991 Assessing schizophrenia in adults with mental retardation. A comparative study. British Journal of Psychiatry 158: 103–105

Moss S, Patel P, Prosser H et al 1993 Psychiatric morbidity in older people with moderate and severe learning disability (mental retardation). Part 1: Development and reliability of the patient interview (the PAS-ADD). British Journal of Psychiatry 163: 471–480

Moss S, Goldberg D, Patel P et al 1996a The psychiatric assessment schedule for adults with a developmental disability: PAS-ADD. Hester Adrian Research Centre, Manchester

Moss S, Prosser H, Goldberg D 1996b Validity of the schizophrenia diagnosis of the Psychiatric Assessment Schedule for Adults with Developmental Disabilities (PAS-ADD). British Journal of Psychiatry 168: 359–367

Moss S, Ibbotson B, Prosser H et al 1997 Validity of the PAS-ADD for detecting psychiatric symptoms in people with learning disability. Social Psychiatry and Psychiatric Epidemiology 32: 344–354

Moss S, Prosser H, Costello H et al 1998 Reliability and validity of the PAS-ADD Checklist for detecting psychiatric disorders in adults with intellectual disability. Journal of Intellectual Disability Research 42(2): 173–183

O'Neill R F, Horner R H, Albin R W et al 1997 Functional analysis and programme development for problem behavior. A practical handbook, 2nd edn. Brooks Cole, California

Paclawskyj T, Matson J, Bamburg J et al 1997 A comparison of the Diagnostic Assessment for the Severely Handicapped-II (DASH-II) and the Aberrant Behaviour Checklist (ABC). Research in Developmental Disabilities 18(4): 289–298

Powell R 2003 Psychometric properties of the Beck Depression Inventory and the Zung Self-rating Depression Scale in adults with mental retardation. Mental Retardation 41(2): 88–95

Prasher V P 1997 Dementia questionnaire for persons with mental retardation: modified criteria for adults with Down's syndrome. Journal of Applied Research in Intellectual Disabilities 10(1): 54–60

Prosser H, Bromley J 1998 Interviewing people with intellectual disabilities. In: Emerson E, Hatton C, Bromley J et al (eds) Clinical psychology and people with intellectual disabilities. Wiley, Chichester, p 99–113

Prosser H, Moss S, Costello H et al 1996 The Mini PAS-ADD: an assessment schedule for the detection of mental health problems in adults with developmental disabilities. Hester Adrian Research Centre, University of Manchester

Prosser H, Moss S, Costello H et al 1998 Reliability and validity of the Mini PAS-ADD for assessing psychiatric disorders in adults with intellectual disability. Journal of Intellectual Disability Research 42(4): 264–272

Raghavan R 2000 Cardinal signs. Learning Disability Practice 3(3): 25–27

Raghavan R, Marshall M, Lockwood A et al 2001 The learning disabilities version of the cardinal needs schedule (LDCNS) (unpublished; available from r.raghavan@bradford.ac.uk)

Reiss S 1994 The Reiss screen for maladaptive behaviour test manual, 2nd edn. IDS Publishing, Worthington, OH

Reiss S, Valenti-Hein D 1994 Development of a psychopathology rating scale for children with mental retardation. Journal of Consulting and Clinical Psychology 62(1): 28–33

Ross E, Oliver C 2003 The assessment of mood in adults who have severe or profound mental retardation. Clinical Psychology Review 23: 234–245

Roy A, Matthews H, Clifford P et al 2002 The Health of the Nation Outcome Scales for people with learning disabilities (HoNOS-LD). Royal College of Psychiatrists, London

Royal College of Psychiatrists 2001 DC-LD (Diagnostic criteria for psychiatric disorders for use with adults with learning disabilities/mental retardation). Occasional Paper OP48. Gaskell, London

Slade M, Thornicroft G, Loftus L et al 1999 The Camberwell Assessment of Need. Gaskell, London

Sturmey P, Reed J, Corbett J 1991 Psychometric assessment of psychiatric disorders in people with learning difficulties (mental handicap): a review of measures. Psychological Medicine 21: 143–155

Tunmore R 2000 Practitioner assessment skills. In: Thompson T, Mathias P (eds) Lyttle's mental health and disorder, 3rd edn. Baillière Tindall, Edinburgh, p 481–496

Wing J K, Curtis R H, Beevor A S 1996 Health of the nation outcome scales. Raters' Pack. Royal College of Psychiatrists College Research Unit, London

World Health Organization 1992 ICD-10: The international statistical classification of diseases and related health problems, 10th revision. WHO, Geneva

World Health Organization 1996 ICD-10 guide for mental retardation. WHO, Geneva

Xenitidis K, Thornicroft G, Leese M et al 2000 Reliability and validity of the CANDID – a needs assessment instrument for adults with learning disabilities and mental health problems. British Journal of Psychiatry 176: 473–478

Zigmond A, Snaith R 1983 The Hospital Anxiety and Depression Scale. Acta Psychiatrica Scandinavica 67: 361–370

Zung W K 1965 A self-rating scale for depression. Archives of General Psychiatry 12: 63–70

Zung W K 1971 A rating instrument for anxiety disorders. Psychosomatics 12: 371–379

7

Therapeutic interventions

INTRODUCTION

This chapter will discuss a range of physical and non-physical therapeutic intervention strategies designed to address mental health problems, and will consider if and how these might be adapted to meet the needs of people with learning disabilities. It should be noted that the majority of interventions described in this chapter require at least a minimum level of training in their use, and that some require specialist training and qualifications. Nonetheless, the therapeutic role of the care worker in contributing to mental health interventions will be explored, and finally, the chapter will discuss consent to treatment for people with learning disabilities.

Finding the appropriate intervention

As we have seen in previous chapters, interest in the mental health needs of people with learning disabilities is a fairly recent phenomenon. Consequently, as Caine & Hatton (1998, p 219) have pointed out, 'the historical neglect of mental health issues…is reflected in a corresponding lack of interest in treatment issues'. Furthermore, there is a view that treatment for people with learning disabilities who experience emotional problems is currently inadequate (Hollins & Sinason 2000). It has been acknowledged that evidence about effective interventions is limited, and what evidence there is has been transferred from adult mental health services, which is not always appropriate or beneficial for people with learning disabilities (Oliver et al 2003).

These views should not surprise us. As we saw in Chapter 2, getting to the root cause of a client's problem is far from straightforward, and there can be many explanations as to why a person is suffering in the way that they are. As we also saw in Chapter 2, the choice of treatment and intervention designed to remove or alleviate symptoms of mental ill health is, for the most part, directly related to the way in which the problem has been understood and explained. So, for example, if we return to the case of Jason introduced in Chapter 2, and decide that his problems stem from having experienced a loss in his life (when his father moved out of the family home), then we might conclude that he would benefit from the opportunity to express the meaning of this loss and, if appropriate, to grieve over it. So we might suggest a 'talking' intervention such as counselling or psychotherapy. If, however, we decide that there does not appear to be a clear trigger for his problems, or if his problems are severe enough to affect his physical functioning, then we might decide that there are some biochemical factors inherent within his problems, and that he might respond best to a physical treatment such as medication or electroconvulsive therapy (ECT). Furthermore, as Jason's mother is finding it difficult to understand and cope with her son's change in behaviour, we might feel that both of them would benefit from some supportive or educational inputs.

Equally, we might decide that Jason and his mum would benefit best from a combination or 'package' of interventions, such as regular medication accompanied by input from a counsellor or attendance at a youth support group, and educative–supportive interventions for his mother. This would be an example of an eclectic approach as described in Chapter 2.

Thus we can see that the process of deciding upon the most appropriate treatment or intervention is not entirely straightforward, and is based upon a careful assessment, accurate diagnosis, and thorough monitoring of the effectiveness of the prescribed intervention. As we saw in Chapter 3, assessing the mental health needs of people with learning disabilities is fraught with difficulties, and without accurate assessment and diagnosis of mental health problems, the identification of the most appropriate intervention is impossible. Consequently the role of direct care staff in contributing to the assessment, diagnosis, and monitoring process cannot be underestimated, for without an appropriate regime to address the mental health problems, the client and family may experience unnecessary or prolonged suffering.

Can mental health problems be cured?

A question that is often asked is: 'Can mental health problems be cured?' In Chapter 1, when we considered the history of the care and treatment of people with learning disabilities, we discovered that by the late 1700s the distinction between learning disability and other 'mental' problems had become widely accepted, with the chief difference being that learning disabilities could never be 'cured'. This distinction has perhaps led to the belief that mental health problems are curable or reversible. This belief is not entirely accurate. Whereas some mental health problems can resolve altogether over time or in response to interventions, and the symptoms and distress caused by many mental health problems can often be alleviated by appropriate intervention, it is not always possible to say with any certainty that the problem will not recur at some future time, or if intervention ceases. It is likely, also, that a history of mental health problems creates a vulnerability or predisposition to a recurrence of problems when faced with stress or life difficulties in the future.

Against this backdrop, it is encouraging to note that there is now a move on the part of clients and organisations to focus on and promote the concept of recovery from mental health problems, rather than to dwell on incapacity and relapse. Furthermore, what really matters is how individuals perceive themselves, and indeed many people do consider themselves to be recovering or recovered from a mental health problem, or able to cope with it with appropriate support (Baker & Strong 2001). The recovery movement is discussed further in Chapter 8.

MENTAL HEALTH INTERVENTIONS

Having discussed the difficulties inherent in selecting the most appropriate intervention package, we will now turn our attention to the range of interventions that are widely available to address mental health problems. We will consider, in each case, the appropriateness of the intervention for people with learning disabilities, and discuss any necessary adaptations, and will also highlight those interventions that may be utilised independently by care staff.

In line with the different models and explanations of mental health problems introduced in Chapter 2, we discuss *physical* interventions (related to the biological or disease model) and *non-physical* (psychological [psychodynamic, behavioural, cognitive, and humanistic] and social) interventions. It could be argued, also, that *mental health promotion* is an intervention that should be delivered to facilitate recovery and meet the needs of mental health service users, carers, and families (Sainsbury Centre 2001). In this book, mental health promotion is addressed separately in Chapter 8.

While it is recognised that *complementary therapies* such as aromatherapy and massage play an important role in enhancing physical and psychological health, and contribute in particular to the alleviation of anxiety, a specific discussion of complementary therapies is beyond the scope of this book. The interested reader is advised to consult more specialised sources (e.g. Gale & Hegarty 2000, Wray & Patton 2003).

PHYSICAL INTERVENTIONS

It should be noted that the term 'physical intervention' is sometimes used to describe means of responding to challenging behaviour through physical force that limits or restricts the movement or mobility of the individual (British Institute of Learning Disabilities [BILD] 2002). While acknowledging that this type of intervention is sometimes necessary, a discussion is outside the scope of this book, and the interested reader is directed towards more specific texts, such as the many helpful guidelines produced by BILD. This section restricts its focus to a discussion of medication and electroconvulsive therapy in relation to mental health problems and learning disabilities.

Medication

Until fairly recently, it was common for people with learning disabilities to be prescribed a range of psychoactive medication, but it is now becoming clear that this was not always based on the best available evidence, and not always in the client's best interests. As Caine & Hatton (1998, p 219) have pointed out:

Traditionally, treatment has been restricted to the indiscriminate use of psychopharmacy for the purpose of social control, with little matching of drugs to diagnosis, monitoring of short and long-term effects, or evaluation of treatment efficacy.

In the past, many people with learning disabilities, and particularly those in institutional care, received some form of psychoactive medication, particularly anti-psychotic drugs, largely for their tranquillising effect rather than for treating specific psychiatric symptoms (Tyrer 2001). Indeed, they would often be prescribed in the absence of a psychiatric diagnosis, and clients would often receive more than one drug of this type. Fortunately, this trend is beginning to be reversed, and medication is beginning to be used appropriately for the treatment of specific mental health problems rather than to sedate or control behaviours.

Medication can, of course, only be prescribed by a medical practitioner, and therefore a detailed discussion of pharmacological preparations is outside the scope of this book. We would refer interested readers to the multidisciplinary *Psychotropic Medication and Developmental Disabilities: the International Consensus Handbook* (Reiss & Aman 1998) for more detailed information. One of the key skills of a care worker, however, is to monitor and report the effects and side effects of prescribed medication, in order for the client's medical practitioner to be sure that the most appropriate treatment has been prescribed. This is particularly important in relation to people with learning disabilities as they may be unable to express or communicate either the therapeutic or adverse effects of prescribed medication.

It is helpful, therefore, to have an understanding of the main categories of drugs which may be prescribed to help mental health problems, and an awareness of some of the key side effects. Anti-depressant and mood stabilising, anti-psychotic, and anxiolytic medications are reviewed in the following sections.

Anti-depressant medication

These include tricyclic drugs, such as amitryptiline and clomipramine, monoamine oxidase inhibitors (MAOIs) such as moclobemide, and selective serotonin reuptake inhibitors (SSRIs) such as fluoxetine (more commonly known as Prozac®). Some anti-depressants, particularly clomipramine and most of the SSRIs and MOAIs, are also indicated for the treatment of obsessive–compulsive disorder. Adverse effects of tricyclics include dry mouth, blurred vision, constipation, and urinary retention, and they are particularly toxic in overdose, while SSRIs can cause headache, nausea, and gastrointestinal disturbances, but are reported to be safer in overdose. Some MAOIs (but not usually moclobemide) can interact with foods containing tyramine (e.g. cheese, meat, yeast extracts) to produce hypertension, headache, and pyrexia, so these foods must be avoided.

It is important for carers to note that anti-depressants can take up to 6 weeks to take effect, and this, coupled with unpleasant adverse effects, sometimes leads people to discontinue their use before they have experienced a therapeutic effect. When they have been taken for 6 weeks or longer, anti-depressants should not normally be stopped abruptly, as this can produce withdrawal effects such as dizziness, anxiety, and mood swings.

While the automatic prescription of drugs for depression in people with learning disabilities is not advised (Tyrer 2001), some case reports show good effects (e.g. Masi et al 1997, Sovner et al 1993). Consensus favours the SSRI anti-depressants, but there are few systematic studies available.

Mood stabilising agents

These are prescribed for the acute treatment and prevention of bipolar affective disorder. The most common drug of this type is lithium, which has many troublesome adverse effects such as thirst, polyuria, tremor, gastrointestinal disturbances, and dermatitis. Regular blood tests are required to ensure therapeutic and not toxic levels.

For people with learning disabilities, lithium may be less effective than in the general population because of the tendency for bipolar disorder in this population to be rapid cycling. When lithium cannot be used or is not effective, anti-epileptic drugs such as carbemazepine and sodium valproate may be useful for people with learning disabilities, as may be the newer anti-epileptics such as lamotrigine, which is particularly indicated for rapid cycling bipolar disorder.

Anti-psychotic medication

These drugs can effectively reduce the symptoms of schizophrenia such as hallucinations and delusions. Some clients, feeling better with medication yet failing to appreciate the need to continue taking it, run a high risk of relapse when these drugs are stopped. For this reason some anti-psychotic drugs can be administered by long-acting depot injection to increase compliance. The older anti-psychotic drugs such as chlorpromazine and haloperidol can produce extrapyramidal side effects (movement disorders), including akathisia (restlessness), dystonia (abnormal movements of the face, eyes, and tongue), pseudo-Parkinsonism (rigidity of the limbs, trunk and neck together with tremor), and tardive dyskinesia (involuntary mouth and jaw movements, sticking out of the tongue, grimacing, shoulder shrugging and rocking movements). Some of these effects can be minimised or prevented by prescribing other drugs known as anti-muscarinic agents, such as procyclidine, as required. Other adverse effects include sedation, weight gain, photosensitivity, and constipation.

Because of these adverse effects, newer 'atypical' anti-psychotic drugs such as risperidone and olanzapine are now more likely to be prescribed for new clients (Taylor et al 2001), as they can be as effective as the older drugs with fewer adverse effects. However, for those clients who have taken the older drugs for some time with no ill effects, there may be little reason to change. For treatment resistant schizophrenia, the atypical drug clozapine may be used, which claims to address both positive and negative symptoms and to reduce the incidence of suicide (Bloye & Davies 1999, Taylor et al 2001). However, although this drug produces fewer extrapyramidal side effects than other anti-psychotics, it can produce a range of adverse effects including weight gain, hypersalivation, sedation, constipation, hypotension, and hypertension, together with risk of the life-threatening condition agranulocytosis. For this reason, regular blood monitoring is required.

Anti-psychotic medication for people with learning disabilities should only be used when there is a clearly defined schizophrenic illness, as there is some evidence that people with organic brain impairments are more likely to develop tardive dyskinesia than the general population (Clarke 2001). Furthermore, there is likely to be a further impairment of cognitive functioning if the dose is high. These drugs also have an effect on convulsive thresholds so there may be additional difficulties if clients have epilepsy. Some studies have reported good effects and fewer side effects with atypical anti-psychotics (e.g. Advokat et al 2000, Williams et al 2000), but at the present time, there is insufficient evidence to judge with confidence the effectiveness of treatment for people with learning disabilities (Duggan & Brylewski 2001).

For those clients who have been inappropriately prescribed anti-psychotic medication, a reduction/withdrawal programme is advocated; Ahmed et al

(2000) showed that a substantial proportion of people with learning disabilities prescribed anti-psychotics for the reduction of behaviour problems can have these drugs safely reduced or withdrawn.

Anxiolytic medication

While the treatment of choice for all anxiety disorders is cognitive–behaviour therapy (Taylor et al 2001; see later in this chapter), anxiolytic drugs may also be prescribed. Examples include diazepam, clonazepam, and the newer buspirone. Drugs such as temazepam are also prescribed for their hypnotic effect for clients with sleep disturbance.

Anxiolytics should only be used in people with learning disabilities for acute anxiety reactions or, if possible, not at all. Prolonged treatment is not recommended as there is a risk of addiction. It is important that medication is gradually withdrawn and not stopped suddenly, as there is a risk of withdrawal seizures. Buspirone is less sedating and has less risk of addiction or withdrawal symptoms, and has been used effectively to treat generalised anxiety in people with learning disabilities. However, there are few research studies into the efficacy of anxiolytic medication in this population (Crabbe 2001).

Electroconvulsive therapy

Electroconvulsive therapy (ECT) has been used since the 1930s, but it is only since the latter part of the 20th century that its use has been restricted primarily to the treatment of severe depression or mania. It is also occasionally used in the treatment of obsessive–compulsive disorder. ECT is normally only administered on an in-patient basis, because prior to administration the client requires a full physical examination, electrocardiogram (ECG) and full blood count, and will receive a short-acting general anaesthetic and a muscle relaxant before the treatment itself is administered. However, it is possible for some people to receive ECT on an out-patient basis.

The treatment itself involves passing a mild electrical current through the brain, via two electrodes placed on the client's head, normally both on one side of the head (unilateral ECT) but occasionally one on each side (bilateral ECT). The size of the current is determined by the client's sex, height, and weight, and the strength of any previous current administered. The electrical current induces an epileptic-type seizure lasting between 15 and 35 seconds, but as the patient has received a muscle-relaxing drug, the effects of the seizure are normally minor; often all that can be seen is a twitching of the toes. Furthermore, as a general anaesthetic has been administered, the client is unaware of the experience. Following the treatment the patient will feel drowsy and will require vigilant observation in a recovery area and for some time afterwards.

Many studies have demonstrated the effectiveness of ECT, and some studies have claimed that it is more effective than medication alone in the treatment of severe depression or mania. Certainly, it can have a faster effect than most of the anti-depressant drugs in common use, because these typically take some weeks for the sufferer to experience any benefit. However, its use is controversial, not least because no-one is absolutely certain how it works, but also because there are likely to be some unpleasant side effects following treatment, such as headache and short-term memory loss. Critics claim that because the long-term effects have not been systematically studied, the treatment should not be used. Supporters would argue that in severe depression or mania, particularly when there is a risk of suicide, it may be the preferred treatment option, as its effects are likely to be much faster than those of medication.

There is little evidence available in relation to the use of ECT with people with learning disabilities. A study carried out by Cutajar & Wilson (1999) in one NHS region in the UK found that only eight people with learning disabilities (from a total population of 4.7 million) had received ECT during the previous 5 years, which is very low in comparison to the number of people receiving ECT in the general population. Ruedrich & Alamir (1999) reviewed 14 case reports describing ECT being used in 20 individuals with learning disabilities, most of which supported its efficacy and safety. In all, the little evidence that is available seems to suggest that the use of ECT with people with learning disabilities can be as safe and effective as with anyone in the general population, and that it can be a useful alternative where patients do not respond to, or are intolerant of, pharmacological treatments. Cutajar & Wilson's (1999) study suggests that best results are obtained when the patient suffers from depression dominated by biological and/or psychotic symptoms. However, most of the studies that have been reported are small-scale case reports rather than systematic studies, and further research is required to test the efficacy and safety of ECT for people with learning disabilities. Furthermore, as informed consent is required before ECT may be administered, there may be some particular difficulties in explaining the treatment and gaining informed consent from people with learning disabilities (see discussion on consent later in this chapter).

NON-PHYSICAL INTERVENTIONS

It could be argued that all non-physical interventions designed to address mental health problems are *psychosocial interventions*, in that they draw upon psychological and/or social knowledge to address problems in this area. In the UK, Hatton's (2002) review of psychosocial interventions for people with learning disabilities includes cognitive–behaviour therapy, psychodynamic psychotherapy, and group intervention as examples. In the USA, Rush & Frances's (2000) consensus guidelines for the treatment of

mental health and behavioural problems for people with learning disabilities lists seven types of intervention under the heading of 'psychosocial
interventions'. These are cognitive–behaviour therapy, supportive counselling, classical behaviour therapy, applied behaviour analysis, psychotherapy, managing the environment, and client and/or family education. All of
these are considered in the following sections.

Psychological interventions: psychodynamic approaches

Psychodynamic treatment methods are directed towards the underlying
problem rather than the symptoms or behaviours. The aim is for clients to
gain insight into their problems and change feelings, cognition and behaviour, through the medium of a therapeutic relationship with the therapist.
Communication between the client and the therapist involves the therapist in
listening, facilitating emotional expression, and making interpretations, with
the aim of identifying unconscious conflicts and transference feelings. The
therapist does not normally give advice but helps the client to work through
unconscious conflicts. For this reason it is most frequently considered a treatment option for problems in which the client retains insight and remains in
touch with reality, such as depression and anxiety, and is rarely considered
suitable for clients with psychotic disorders such as schizophrenia.

The most well-known psychodynamic interventions are individual or
group psychotherapy, although some forms of creative therapy (e.g. art,
drama, music therapy) are based on psychodynamic principles.

Individual psychotherapy

The emphasis of individual psychotherapy is on resolving unconscious
conflicts, through the use of transference and counter-transference in the
therapeutic relationship. *Transference* occurs when the client unconsciously
transfers onto the therapist positive or negative feelings associated with
relationships with other people, such as family members. Transference is
used by the therapist to understand and interpret the inner world of the
client. *Counter-transference* is the therapist's reactions to the client, and the
therapist must acknowledge and work through such feelings in the course
of the relationship.

Group therapy

There are many forms of group therapy; groups can be primarily supportive, task focused, or therapeutic. The principle behind group psychotherapy is that the group should be centred on itself rather than on the leader,
and as with individual therapy, transference and counter-transference

occurring between members and the leader will be explored. Group dynamics, i.e. patterns of behaviour occurring within the group, are explored, and the group's awareness of verbal and non-verbal communication can be enhanced. Individual members may be enabled to explore and accept their limitations, and improve their social interaction and interpersonal relationships (Hollins 2001).

Creative therapies

The use of creative therapies (art, music, dance, poetry, and drama) can be particularly useful when verbal language is not available. In addition to having a therapeutic role, these activities can provide recreation and leisure or be used for remedial purposes, where they are planned by a therapist to help a client work towards a pre-set goal or objective. As therapy, however, what they have in common is active rather than passive participation, together with an emphasis on the process rather than on the creation of a specific end product (Reynolds 1999). The therapeutic relationship is the key tool, as it is with the talking psychotherapies. Equally, creative therapies can be carried out with individuals or within groups. Some therapists aim to interpret the messages communicated through the various media in a meaningful way, but as with talking therapies, this level of intervention will require training. Even when this level of interpretation is not required, creative therapies can be therapeutic as they allow for the expression of needs and positive and negative emotions in a safe and structured environment. They can facilitate non-verbal channels of communication, and promote positive self-image and self-esteem, by allowing clients to try out new skills and roles, and obtain feedback (Reynolds 1999).

Psychotherapy and people with learning disabilities

Perhaps because of the need to explore deep rooted and often unconscious conflicts, psychotherapies have in the past been infrequently used with people with learning disabilities. The first case reported was of a 33-year-old man with an IQ of 59 who attended a day centre (Symington 1981). This reluctance to use psychotherapy may stem from the ideas of Freud, who suggested that 'those patients who do not possess a reasonable degree of education and reliable character should be refused [psychotherapy]', thus perpetuating the erroneous assumptions that people with learning disabilities do not have the intellectual capacity to experience or express mental distress, or the ability to develop insight because of their level of intelligence (Caine & Hatton 1998). Indeed, in the past, emotional experiences may have been discounted because people with learning disabilities have not been encouraged to talk about how they feel, and may instead have expressed their emotions through a range of behaviours such as aggression.

It is now recognised that people with learning disabilities experience emotional difficulties in relation to loss, grieving, bonding, attachment, separation, rejection, anticipation of failure, fear, and inadequacy (Arthur 2003). Emotional responses to these difficulties may manifest themselves as challenging behaviour and not be understood by carers. While it is acknowledged that some people with learning disabilities have difficulties in recognising the expression of emotions in others, so too do many people without learning disabilities (Arthur 2003). This does not mean that they experience difficulties in expressing emotions, even when they have severe and profound levels of disability.

Hollins (2001) suggests that there are several key areas of difficulty or 'secrets' that people with learning disabilities typically experience, and which they are likely to bring to individual or group therapy if given the opportunity. These are the disability itself, loss, dependency, and sexuality. Although for many people with and without a learning disability, talking about emotions is difficult, Gravestock (1995) argues that some people with learning disabilities may be more ready to share feelings than people with normal intelligence because they may lack some defence mechanisms. Furthermore, many have positive personality traits including the capacity to survive, forgive, and maintain a sense of humour, all of which are useful in a psychotherapeutic context. In differentiating between cognitive or 'thinking' intelligence and emotional or 'feeling' intelligence, Hodges (2003) suggests that although people with learning disabilities may lack the former, emotional intelligence may develop age-appropriately, and to some extent such individuals may have a deep emotional capacity and be well able to get in touch with emotions.

While transference may be different in people with learning disabilities, especially if they have a limited vocabulary through which to express it, nevertheless it is possible to focus on wordless expressions of feelings (Hodges 2003). Indeed, it has been noted that as therapy is not an intellectual activity, then cognitive ability is irrelevant when considering someone's suitability for therapy (Esterhuyzen & Hollins 1997), and that all that is required of a person with learning disabilities to benefit from psychotherapy is the ability to make emotional contact and forge a relationship with the therapist (Hollins 2001).

Challenges to using psychotherapy with people with learning disabilities

There remain, however, considerable challenges to the use of psychotherapies with people with learning disabilities. Apart from the fact that there are, and are always likely to be, inadequate numbers of experienced and trained therapists and services (Arthur 2003), psychotherapy implies, as we have seen, an intimate, confiding, and often long-term relationship. It may be difficult to ensure the appropriate conditions of privacy and confidentiality, especially if the person lives within a close-knit family unit, or in an institution or group-based residence where all activities are normally shared with other clients and caregivers (Hollins 2001).

As with any therapy, there may be difficulties in achieving informed consent, and techniques may need adaptations to suit the intellectual ability of the client. For example, pictorial aids may be helpful to facilitate the exploration of emotions. Termination of therapy – whether individual, group, or creative – has to be particularly sensitively handled so as not to reinforce any previous experiences of loss or rejection. The process is likely to place considerable emotional demands upon the therapist and intensive supervision is required. Furthermore, it is difficult, as with any therapeutic intervention, to draw firm conclusions about outcomes, and there is a paucity of evidence in relation to outcomes of psychotherapy with people with learning disabilities (Beail 1995, Kelly 2001). In the early case recorded by Symington (1981), for example, after 2 years of therapy, the client was more able to express his feelings, but became less cooperative with staff. Is this evidence of a successful outcome, or not? Similar studies that have been reported are of the single case study variety (Hodges 2003), making it difficult to draw generalisable conclusions.

Evidence is now beginning to emerge, however, about the effectiveness of psychotherapeutic interventions for people with learning disabilities (e.g. Beail 1995, 1998), including those with severe or profound levels of disability (Sinason 1992), and continued research and staff training are needed to ensure that people with learning disabilities are not denied access to a range of approaches that may be of enormous therapeutic benefit.

Psychological interventions: behavioural approaches

In contrast to the psychotherapies, behavioural approaches operate by focusing on and aiming to change or modify observable behaviours, or symptoms, rather than deal with the inner or unconscious feelings that might be causing them. They will be very familiar to many care workers in the field of learning disabilities. Until at least the 1980s, behavioural treatment approaches were commonly used and many practitioners, particularly nurses, were trained to use predominantly behavioural strategies in their day-to-day work. This is perhaps unsurprising given the erroneous belief that people with learning disabilities did not have the mental capacity or intellect to gain insight into the root causes of their difficulties.

Perhaps less popular in mental health care, nonetheless behavioural interventions were frequently used, and for a period of time in the 1970s approaches based on behavioural principles such as the token economy scheme were popular in mental health settings. In such schemes, 'tokens' which could be exchanged for personal items such as sweets or cosmetics were issued as a reward for desirable behaviour.

As we saw in Chapter 2, behavioural approaches are based on the theories of learning devised by psychologists such as Pavlov (1849–1936), Skinner (1904–1990), and Bandura (1925–) in the early part of the 20th century. Pavlov's theory of classical conditioning can be described as *learning by association*. He postulated that we build up new learning when two previously unassociated ideas become linked together. Sometimes, learning is faulty because ideas that should not be associated with one another do in fact become associated, such as the sight of a spider and a fear response. Classical conditioning, therefore, is the basis of some treatments for phobias and obsessional disorders, and aims to reverse this faulty association process.

Skinner's theory of operant conditioning can be described as *learning by consequences* and is the basis of behaviour modification and programmes such as the token economy system. The aim is to increase desirable behaviours through manipulating the consequences of that behaviour, such that the client learns to behave in the desired way in the future. Manipulation might involve, for example, praising a client's efforts to decorate their room, but ignoring (within the boundaries of health and safety) the mess made in the process.

Within mental health care, it is perhaps the work of Pavlov that has had most impact in that it led to the development of a range of interventions based on breaking the association between two things that had become linked through faulty learning. In the early days, techniques were used that would be questionable on ethical grounds today, such as attempting to remove sexually deviant behaviour by showing people films or pictures of such activity while at the same time administering a mild electric shock. Equally, the once popular treatment for alcoholism, which involved administering a drug which, if followed by drinking alcohol, would cause the individual to feel extremely physically ill, is, even with informed consent, ethically questionable.

However, there is still a place for classical conditioning approaches such as in the treatment of phobias. A phobia is an irrational fear of an object or situation that generally leads to avoidance of that object or situation. While it might be fairly easy for most people to avoid heights, or spiders, it is much more difficult to avoid situations such as using public transport, shopping, or socialising with others, the fear of which may have arisen through faulty associative learning in the past. The aim of therapy would be to expose the individual gradually to the object of their fears while supporting and helping them to relax through the exposure. In this way, the faulty association between the feared object or situation and the fear itself should, over a period of time, weaken and eventually disappear. This is known as systematic desensitisation. In the past, more drastic approaches to breaking the association were used, where, for example, the individual would be exposed to their worst fear, the idea being that if they could prove to themselves that no harm had come to them, they need no longer fear the object or situation. However, this approach, known as flooding, is infrequently used today.

Behavioural interventions can also be used with good effect in obsessive–compulsive disorders, by exposing the client to real ('in vivo') situations that are likely to activate compulsive behaviour, but then preventing the client from carrying out these compulsions, such that they learn that they are able to resist compulsions without adverse effects.

There is a range of other interventions drawing upon the behavioural model to address client mental health difficulties. These include problem solving, relaxation, modelling, assertiveness training, and anger management. As most of these have a cognitive as well as a behavioural component, they are considered under cognitive interventions in the following section.

The question that still remains, however, if we change behaviour but do not address its underlying cause, is whether the problem will still exist, and manifest itself as another undesirable behaviour in the future. Although there is little evidence available to prove that this actually happens following a behavioural intervention, nevertheless it may be most helpful to offer clients a package of interventions, such that they can be free from undesirable symptoms or behaviours, while at the same time being encouraged to talk about and understand how these symptoms might have arisen in the first place.

Psychological interventions: cognitive approaches

While the behavioural approach developed in an attempt to make the explanation of, and treatment for, behavioural problems more scientific, there soon developed a view that the approach was limited in scope and could not explain or address every type of problem, particularly those involving thinking, reasoning, or problem-solving. As discussed in Chapter 2, the cognitive model began as a form of treatment, initially for depression, and is based on the idea that mental health problems are caused by errors in thinking. In other words, how we think determines how we feel. It follows, therefore, that if faulty thinking and belief systems can be challenged, the associated behavioural and emotional problems will decrease or disappear. Cognitive therapy addresses an individual's negative thoughts and beliefs, and has been shown to be as effective as medication in the general population (Ruedrich et al 2001).

Cognitive–behaviour therapy

As discussed in Chapter 2, while cognitive therapy alone became popular for a while, more often today it is combined with behavioural interventions to produce a range of cognitive–behavioural therapies. Probably the most well known and widely used intervention that draws upon the cognitive explanation of mental ill health is cognitive–behaviour therapy (CBT). Although CBT is not a single therapy, but is a generic term for many different therapies, the approach has been advocated as the treatment of choice for numerous psychological and mental health problems (Department of Health 1999). It has made a significant contribution in the general population, in particular for the treatment of depression, or following trauma or abuse (Hollins & Sinason 2000), in stress and anxiety (Taylor et al 2001), and in psychosis (Drury 2000, Fahy & Dudley 2000). It claims to be effective by tackling both the symptoms and the underlying problems, and in helping clients to recognise the 'vicious circles' that maintain problems, to challenge negative thoughts and to re-frame them in a more positive light, such that, for example, 'I am a failure' becomes 'I was unsuccessful in that job interview because I did not prepare fully for it, but in other areas of my life, such as looking after my children, I am successful'.

Cognitive–behavioural interventions are also highly effective as part of the treatment package for schizophrenia, and in particular in helping clients to deal with the distressing symptoms of hallucinations and delusions. For example, clients can be encouraged to focus on auditory hallucinations (voices), describe the characteristics of the voices and what they say, describe their thoughts about the voices, and then challenge these thoughts. In other words, they are helped to view the voices as their own thoughts, and so to challenge them, resulting in less distress. Similarly, CBT can be used to help clients to express and challenge delusional ideas (Fahy & Dudley 2000).

Other cognitive–behavioural interventions

There is a range of other interventions drawing upon the behavioural, cognitive and to some extent social models which aim to address specific client mental health difficulties. Most learning disability care workers will be familiar with *social skills training*, which aims to shape behaviour towards performance of a desired skill or group of skills by breaking them down into small components, allowing the client to observe and practise each component until a level of skill has been achieved, and at the same time providing feedback and positive reinforcement such as praise from the carer.

Problem solving guides clients towards a range of problem solutions and helps them to visualise and consider the consequences of each. In some cases, the therapist or carer can role-play possible solutions and encourage the client to practise the solutions they have observed (Benson & Valenti-Hein 2001). This element of problem solving draws upon Bandura's social learning theory, and is based on the idea that we learn through observing and sometimes imitating behaviours of other people, who serve as role models, particularly if we see these role models themselves being rewarded for their actions. Consequently care workers have a huge responsibility in acting as positive role models to their clients, both in their everyday actions and interactions, and in specific situations where a change in behaviour is desirable.

Other cognitively focused interventions include reality orientation and reminiscence therapy. *Reality orientation* uses environmental changes such as prompts, aids, and reminders to promote and restore the orientation of the individual in relation to time, place, and person. Signs, calendars, notice boards, and pictures can all be used to good effect, as can general communication strategies such as using short, specific sentences, commenting on current events, referring to clients' past experiences, and constantly using reminders of who the person is, where the person is, and the time of day, month, season, or year. Reality orientation should be a 24-hour basic informal communication approach, but can also be used within structured group sessions.

Reminiscence therapy is an approach in which the natural inclination of individuals to return past experiences to consciousness is fostered in order to improve sense of identity, self-esteem, mood, communication skills, cognitive skills, problem solving and coping strategies (Hseih & Wang 2003). Again, reminiscence can be carried out during everyday interactions with clients, but can also be used within formal structured group sessions using a range of prompts and artefacts relating to clients' histories to stimulate past memories. The creation and use of life books, in addition to promoting the identity and individuality of clients, can also stimulate memories and enhance the maintenance of cognitive function.

Anger management, relaxation training, and assertiveness training are all related in some way to the behavioural and cognitive models of intervention, and their use with people with learning disabilities is discussed below.

Cognitive–behaviour therapies and people with learning disabilities

Until recently cognitive–behaviour therapies had not received much interest for people with learning disabilities because of the idea that they could not explore personal meaning (Stenfert Kroese 1997), but evidence of the benefits is beginning to emerge. Lindsay et al (1993), for example, described the successful use of group cognitive therapy for people with learning disabilities who were suffering from depression. Within this approach, there are several stages based on the aim of establishing a relationship between thoughts, feelings, and behaviour:

1. An agenda is set.
2. Negative thoughts are isolated.
3. Underlying assumptions are elicited.
4. The group aims to test the accuracy of thinking and to generate alternative positive ways of thinking, through the development of

reflective skills and through encouraging participants to offer positive thoughts to their peers.

5. Monitoring thoughts and feelings may be facilitated through the use of visual analogue scales and role play.

At the end of every group, homework is set whereby clients identify negative thoughts and suggest how they might change these into positive ones, using daily diaries if appropriate.

Lindsay et al (1997) also described the effective use of cognitive–behaviour therapy for people with learning disabilities who have anxiety.

Howells et al (2000) described the effective use of a group cognitive–behavioural approach for *anger management*, although it was not possible to measure outcomes conclusively. Clients were taught first:

- to recognise feelings in others
- to recognise physical and emotional signs of anger in themselves
- to become aware of triggers to their anger
- to consider reasons why people might become angry
- to appreciate the consequences of becoming angry.

Following this, clients were taught alternatives to physical and verbal aggression when they felt angry, such as assertiveness, negotiation, and problem solving. Role play and video work were incorporated into the sessions.

Rose et al (2000) also used these techniques within group interventions for anger that included relaxation, self-instruction, and problem solving. A significant feature was that a care worker accompanied each client to the groups, thus making them more accessible for a range of disability levels. Not only did the sessions reduce anger, they also reduced reported levels of depression in the client group.

Cognitive–behavioural approaches are inherent within interventions such as relaxation therapy and assertiveness training. *Relaxation therapy* focuses on reducing anxiety and is often included as part of anger and anxiety management programmes. There are several techniques available, but most focus on teaching deep breathing techniques together with progressive muscle relaxation, focusing on tensing and relaxing each group of muscles in turn, such that the client can experience and appreciate the difference between muscular tension and relaxation. Once a state of physical relaxation has been achieved, mental relaxation can be encouraged by helping clients to focus on pleasant images and experiences, sometimes accompanied by relaxing music. These techniques, once learned, can be applied in any anxiety-provoking situation or simply to enhance physical and emotional well-being.

Relaxation therapy may need to be adapted for some people with learning disabilities, and particularly for those with more severe disabilities. For example, modelling may be required to demonstrate breathing techniques, or physical guidance may be necessary to help clients to distinguish between tense and relaxed muscles (Lindsay et al 1989).

Assertiveness training helps individuals to communicate their needs and wants clearly, such that their rights are upheld, while not denying the rights of others. Being assertive is a more effective way of communicating needs than by being passive, manipulative or aggressive, and often employs the strategies of negotiation and compromise. Techniques such as modelling and role play can be used to enhance assertive communication in a range of everyday situations such as asking for information, making a complaint, or saying 'no'.

It has been noted that people with learning disabilities, particularly those who have spent time in institutions, have difficulty in communicating their needs assertively as they have often been disempowered in their day-to-day activities and choices. Nezu et al (1991) studied the effects of assertiveness and problem solving training for people with mild learning disabilities; both were effective in reducing mental health symptoms and distress, and in improving anger control, problem solving, and coping skills.

Despite the emerging evidence that people with learning disabilities can benefit from cognitive therapeutic approaches, this requires much more research (Ruedrich et al 2001). Indeed, there are limitations to the use of these types of intervention with people with learning disabilities. Hatton (2002) suggests that in order to be assessed as suitable for cognitive–behaviour therapy, clients must possess a certain level of communication skills, cognitive aptitude, capacity to identify emotions, and capacity to understand the CBT model, hence it is likely to be of most benefit to people at the higher end of the ability level. It is thought that most clients at mild levels of disability can, with help, carry out self-monitoring of thoughts and carry out homework tasks (Ruedrich et al 2001). However, Benson & Valenti-Hein (2001) suggest that, with adaptations, cognitive therapies can be suitable for non-verbal persons or those with more severe intellectual impairments. Certainly, many of the wide range of interventions such as relaxation therapy can be used effectively with people with all levels of learning disabilities.

Psychological interventions: humanistic approaches

Person-centred counselling

Probably the most well known and widely used therapeutic intervention based on the humanistic approach is person-centred counselling, arising out of the work of Carl Rogers (1902–1987). While there are many overlaps between counselling and psychotherapy, person-centred counselling is based on the assumption that individuals will develop in emotionally healthy directions, given the appropriate therapeutic climate (Prout & Cale 1994). The task of the person acting as counsellor is to facilitate an appropriate therapeutic climate which will stimulate emotional growth; this form of counselling is sometimes referred to as non-directive counselling.

Rogers (1961) identified a set of core conditions that he claimed were necessary and sufficient on the part of the counsellor to bring about therapeutic change in the client. These were congruence, unconditional positive regard, and empathy.

- *Congruence*, or genuineness, is a state of being of the counsellor in which what the counsellor says and does matches what he or she thinks and feels (Tschudin 1995).
- *Unconditional positive regard* is a total acceptance and valuing of the individual (positive regard), regardless of the client's background, beliefs or behaviours (unconditional regard).
- *Empathy* is an attempt to enter the emotional world of the client, and so see things from the client's rather than the counsellor's perspective.

These qualities can be communicated both verbally and non-verbally. Empathy, for example, can be communicated verbally through paraphrasing (putting in one's own words) the content of what has been communicated, and making a tentative reflection of the client's feelings. For example, having listened to a client's story of an argument with her mother, the counsellor might say 'So, you had a row with mum on Friday' (paraphrasing the content), 'and it sounds as though you're still feeling angry with her today' (reflecting feelings). If what the client feels is not anger but something else, then this tentative reflection will give the client the opportunity to clarify.

However, empathy can also be communicated effectively through non-verbal means: by sitting at the client's level, leaning towards the client, mirroring the client's posture and movements, by the sensitive use of touch, and by sharing silences. All of these actions communicate a desire to be 'with' the client and to try to understand how it is for them at the moment. Indeed, empathy may be more effectively communicated non-verbally than with words, regardless of whether or not the client has verbal communication skills.

The process of person-centred counselling, then, can be summarised as creating an emotional climate, communicating the core conditions of congruence, empathy and unconditional positive regard, and using active listening, paraphrasing, reflecting emotions, clarifying and summarising, such that the client and counsellor arrive at a shared understanding of the client's situation, and can begin to explore future options and decisions.

Validation therapy

A specialised form of intervention that, like counselling, aims to facilitate the expression of emotion, is *validation therapy* (Feil 2002). This is a means of valuing, through communication, the emotional experiences of older people who have become cognitively impaired. It has some connections with person-centred counselling in that it allows clients to express their emotions freely and for these emotions to be validated and supported by carers. So, for example, if an older person in hospital suffering from Alzheimer's disease is anxiously trying to find her way out of the hospital, as she thinks her mother will be wondering why she is late home from school, rather than try to reorientate her in time and place, as with reality orientation, we would focus on her distress and worry, validate those emotions, and encourage the client to talk about her childhood and her mother. In this way the client's self-worth and interaction skills are promoted, and withdrawal from the outside world is reduced.

Feil (2002) claims that the techniques are simple for carers to learn and can take only a few minutes per day; hence they could be very suitable for carers to use with people with learning disabilities and Alzheimer's disease. The results of observational studies suggest positive effects, although more research is needed (Neal & Briggs 2003).

Counselling and people with learning disabilities

In that person-centred counselling relies on a genuine and unconditional acceptance of the client, it is eminently suitable for people with learning disabilities who may have experienced negative attitudes and responses in the past, including those with limited or absent verbal skills. The techniques of counselling can be used successfully with people with learning disabilities, although initially it may be necessary to provide more direction and focus within sessions than would be usual in general counselling sessions. As with all 'talking' therapies, attention to developmentally appropriate language will be necessary, and the use of supportive materials (such as drawing or games) may be appropriate (Prout & Cale 1994).

While formal counselling requires extensive training and supervision in practice, it is argued that all health and social care professionals can and should use counselling skills in their everyday work, offering time, attention, active listening and an honest, empathic and non-judgemental approach, in order to build self-esteem, self-worth, and autonomy within their clients.

Social interventions

We have already noted, in Chapter 2, a range of interventions such as family therapy, which focus on social and environmental change in order to produce therapeutic benefits. The effects upon family members of having a relative with learning disabilities and associated mental health problems are discussed further in Chapter 10. While good practice dictates that wherever possible, family members or significant others will be involved in all decisions about treatment for clients with learning disabilities who also have mental health problems, some interventions specifically engage family members within the therapeutic process.

Family therapy

Structured approaches to family involvement are sometimes helpful when an individual family member's problems seem to be related to dysfunctional behaviour and communication within the family itself. Family therapy is based on the idea that the behaviour of individuals within families is influenced and maintained by interactions between these family members and with other individuals and systems (Association for Family Therapy 2003). Thus, rather than focusing on the individual with a problem, the whole family is seen as 'the client', and is assessed to try to discover and address the family dynamics that might be causing individual family members, or the family as a whole, to experience problems.

Although there are a number of different models of family therapy (including structural, strategic, and systemic), what most approaches have in common is the requirement that the family takes responsibility for itself, and develops a set of rules and strategies for changing dysfunctional behaviour. Family therapy is normally a more directive intervention than psychotherapy (Hollins 2001).

Family interventions in psychosis

Although, as we have seen, we now have effective medication for controlling or reducing the severity of symptoms in mental health problems such as schizophrenia and bipolar disorder, it seems that medication alone is inadequate to prevent relapse. It is known that a high percentage of people discharged following treatment for psychosis without additional support and intervention will suffer a relapse in the following year. However, it is not simply the presence of support that reduces the risk of relapse; it is the quality of that support that is significant. Research carried out during the 1970s began to show that clients who had been treated successfully for mental health problems, notably schizophrenia, and who returned to live within family environments where there was high emotional involvement, hostility and criticism (described as 'high expressed emotion' environments), were much more likely to relapse than those returning to 'low expressed emotion' environments (Brown et al 1972, Vaughan & Leff 1976). Family intervention studies have subsequently shown that high expressed emotion is a good predictor of relapse, and that it is possible to reduce this risk if appropriate anti-psychotic medication is combined with effective family-based interventions, the keys to which are family education, early recognition, and early intervention.

Family education is important in that if families can learn about symptoms and how to respond to them, they are less likely to be critical and pressurising, and consequently the degree of stress in the environment is likely to reduce. Thus clients and their families can be taught simple distraction techniques to deal with hallucinations and delusions, such as using a personal stereo to block out 'voices', or more structured cognitive–behavioural interventions that will help clients themselves to challenge voices or delusional ideas. Furthermore, an understanding of the nature of negative symptoms will help families to recognise that the client is not just being lazy or difficult.

Additionally, it is known that the longer the time taken to obtain treatment, the poorer the outcome (Fahy & Dudley 2000). Hence if clients and families can be taught to identify the signs that indicate the onset of a psychotic episode (known as 'prodromal symptoms'), such as sleep changes, feelings of anxiety, or poor concentration, and then to monitor systematically for the presence of these early signs and prepare a plan of action to seek help (early intervention) when they are noted, relapse may be prevented (Van Meijel et al 2002).

There is now considerable evidence pointing to the benefits, within the general population, of family interventions in the prevention and treatment of psychosis. This, together with an increasing confidence that preventive interventions are both realistic and effective (McGorry 2000), has led to the development of specialised early intervention services (Edwards et al 2000).

Family interventions and people with learning disabilities

Despite convincing evidence within the general population, there is little research evidence available regarding the use of family and psychosocial interventions for people with learning disabilities (Hatton 2002). While early interventions, advice, and support are likely to be crucial in reducing the incidence and severity of mental health problems (Day 2001), much more research is needed, particularly in relation to the wide variety of environments in which many people with learning disabilities live, and where 'family' members living in the same household may share no blood or emotional ties with one another.

CONSENT TO TREATMENT

We have discussed in this chapter a wide range of therapeutic interventions for mental health problems, and have considered their use for people with learning disabilities. These interventions have ranged from highly invasive procedures, such as ECT, to more gentle and supportive measures such as person-centred counselling. However, no matter what form the intervention takes, no intervention should ever be instigated with people with learning disabilities without gaining their consent.

Practitioners have a legal duty to explain the benefits and possible risks of a proposed intervention, what it involves, the implications of not having the

treatment, and any alternatives, even if this ⁚
asked for. The recipient of this information i⸱
treatment, even if this is clearly against th⸱

The Department of Health (2001) disᵕ
between people who have the capacity to coᵢ
For those who have the capacity to consent, wᵕ
people with learning disabilities, they must be able to coᵢ ᵢ
use in decision making the information that is being proviᵤ
must be provided with enough information in an appropriate
able to make the decision to consent. Consent thus obtained should ᵥ
(i.e. the individual must be capable of making the decision) and they shoᵤ
be acting voluntarily, although good practice would dictate that carers and
families should be involved in the discussions. In all cases, it should be
made clear that their decision is not 'for all time'; they have the right to
change their mind in the future.

Unless subject to certain sections of the Mental Health Act (1983), clients
are entitled to refuse any proposed treatment. The Mental Health Act (1983)
can only authorise compulsory treatment of a mental disorder for people
detained under Section 2 (assessment) or Section 3 (treatment) of the Act.
Under proposals to reform the Act (Department of Health 2000, 2002), there
will be a three-stage process to determine whether compulsory treatment
is indicated, set within the context of the Human Rights Act (1998). The
Mental Health Act also allows for a second opinion by an appointed doctor
if the person is deemed incompetent to understand and therefore to consent
to treatment.

Many people with learning disabilities can make informed choices when
given appropriate information about possible risks. However, the situation
is more difficult when the client has a more severe learning disability, and
may not have the capacity to consent. If a person is unable by reason of
mental disability to understand or retain information about the consequence of making a particular decision, or is unable to make or communicate a decision, that person is deemed to be without capacity. For these
people, such consent can never be obtained from another individual on
their behalf. A decision to treat is then based upon what is in the individual's 'best interests', which include social and psychological benefits as well
as medical benefits.

The concept of 'best interests' makes it lawful to give a treatment to
someone who cannot consent provided that such an action would generally
be agreed upon by a reasonable body of medical practitioners within
the field. As a last resort only, if those responsible for making decisions cannot decide what is in the client's best interests, then the case can be referred
to the courts for a decision. However, for most of the interventions
described in this chapter, it is unlikely that these extreme measures would
be needed.

LUSION

s chapter we have reviewed a range of mental health interventions considered their suitability for people with learning disabilities. As er, of course, each person with learning disabilities and associated mental health problems will need an individual approach based on a detailed assessment of their unique needs, set within the context in which they live. With this in mind, you might, at this point, consider the case studies of Jason, Geoff, Jenny and David introduced so far, and think about the types of intervention that might be appropriate in each case. It is likely, however, that no one intervention will address all their needs, and that an eclectic approach will be required.

In Chapter 8 we explore the role of mental health promotion in enhancing the lives of people with learning disabilities.

REFERENCES

Advokat C, Mayville E, Matson J 2000 Side effect profiles of atypical antipsychotics, typical antipsychotics, or no psychotropic medications in persons with mental retardation. Research in Developmental Disabilities 21: 75–84

Ahmed Z, Fraser W, Kerr M et al 2000 Reducing anti-psychotic medication in people with a learning disability. British Journal of Psychiatry 176: 42–46

Arthur A R 2003 The emotional lives of people with learning disability. British Journal of Learning Disabilities 31: 25–30

Association for Family Therapy and Systemic Practice in the UK 2003 What is family therapy? Online. Available: http://www.aft.org.uk

Baker S, Strong S 2001 Roads to recovery. Mind (National Association for Mental Health), London

Beail N 1995 Outcome of psychoanalysis, psychoanalytic and psychodynamic psychotherapy in people with intellectual disabilities: a review. Changes 13: 186–191

Beail N 1998 Psychoanalytic psychotherapy with men with intellectual disabilities. A preliminary outcome study. British Journal of Medical Psychology 71: 1–11

Benson B, Valenti-Hein D 2001 Cognitive and social learning treatments. In: Došen A, Day K (eds) Treating mental illness and behavior disorders in children and adults with mental retardation. American Psychiatric Press, Washington, p 101–118

Bloye D, Davies S 1999 Psychiatry. Mosby, London

British Institute of Learning Disabilities 2002 Physical interventions: the BILD directory. BILD Publications, Kidderminster

Brown G, Birley J, Wing J 1972 Influence of family life on the course of schizophrenic disorders: a replication. British Journal of Psychiatry 121: 241–258

Caine A, Hatton C 1998 Working with people with mental health problems. In: Emerson E, Hatton C, Bromley J et al (eds) Clinical psychology and people with intellectual disabilities. Wiley, Chichester, p 210–223

Clarke D J 2001 Treatment of schizophrenia. In: Došen A, Day K (eds) Treating mental illness and behavior disorders in children and adults with mental retardation. American Psychiatric Press, Washington, p 183–200

Crabbe H 2001 Treatment of anxiety in persons with mental retardation. In: Došen A, Day K (eds) Treating mental illness and behavior disorders in children and adults with mental retardation. American Psychiatric Press, Washington, p 227–241

Cutajar P, Wilson D 1999 The use of ECT in intellectual disability. Journal of Intellectual Disability Research 43(5): 421–427

Day K 2001 Treatment. An integrative approach. In: Došen A, Day K (eds) Treating mental illness and behavior disorders in children and adults with mental retardation. American Psychiatric Press, Washington, p 519–528

Department of Health 1999 Treatment choice in psychological therapies and counselling: evidence based clinical practice guidelines. Department of Health, London

Department of Health 2000 Reforming the Mental Health Act. Department of Health, London

Department of Health 2001 Seeking consent: working with people with learning disabilities. Department of Health, London

Department of Health 2002 Draft Mental Health Bill. The Stationery Office, London

Drury V 2000 Cognitive behaviour therapy in early psychosis. In: Birchwood M, Fowler D, Jackson C (eds) Early intervention in psychosis. Wiley, Chichester, p 185–212

Duggan L, Brylewski J 2001 Antipsychotic medication for those with both schizophrenia and learning disability (Cochrane Review). In: The Cochrane Library, Issue 1. Update Software, Oxford

Edwards J, McGorry P, Pennell K 2000 Models of early intervention in psychosis: an analysis of service approaches. In: Birchwood M, Fowler D, Jackson C (eds) Early intervention in psychosis. Wiley, Chichester, p 281–314

Esterhuyzen A, Hollins S 1997 Psychotherapy. In: Read S (ed) Psychiatry in learning disability. W B Saunders, London, p 332–349

Fahy K, Dudley M 2000 An introduction to psychosocial interventions in services. In: Thompson T, Mathias P (eds) Lyttle's mental health and disorder. Harcourt, London, p 235–251

Feil N 2002 The validation breakthrough: simple techniques for communicating with people with Alzheimer's-type dementia, 2nd edn. Health Professions Press, Baltimore

Gale E, Hegarty J 2000 The use of touch in caring for people with learning disability. British Journal of Developmental Disabilities 46(2): 97–108

Gravestock S 1995 Individual family and social adjustment. In: Holt G, Kon Y, Bouras N (eds) Mental health in learning disabilities. Pavilion, Brighton, p 15–22

Hatton C 2002 Psychosocial interventions for adults with intellectual disabilities and mental health problems: a review. Journal of Mental Health 11(4): 357–373

Hodges S 2003 Counselling adults with learning disabilities. Palgrave, Basingstoke

Hollins S 2001 Psychotherapeutic methods. In: Došen A, Day K (eds) Treating mental illness and behavior disorders in children and adults with mental retardation. American Psychiatric Press, Washington, p 27–44

Hollins S, Sinason V 2000 Psychotherapy, learning disabilities and trauma: new perspectives. British Journal of Psychiatry 176: 37–41

Howells P, Rogers C, Wilcock S 2000 Evaluating a cognitive/behavioural approach to teaching anger management skills to adults with learning disabilities. British Journal of Learning Disabilities 28: 137–142

Hseih H-F, Wang J-J 2003 Effects of reminiscence therapy on depression in older adults: a systematic review. International Journal of Nursing Studies 40: 335–345

Human Rights Act 1998 The Stationery Office, London

Kelly J 2001 Non-behavioural psychotherapy with people with learning disabilities: equal access to equal benefit? Mental Health Care 4(5): 162–165

Lindsay W, Baty F, Mitchie A et al 1989 A comparison of anxiety treatments with adults who have moderate and severe mental retardation. Research in Developmental Disabilities 10: 129–140

Lindsay W, Howells L, Pitcaithly D 1993 Cognitive therapy for depression with individuals with intellectual disabilities. British Journal of Medical Psychology 66(2): 135–141

Lindsay W, Neilson C, Lawrenson H 1997 Cognitive behaviour therapy for anxiety in people with learning disabilities. In: Stenfert Kroese B, Dagnan D, Loumidis K (eds) Cognitive behaviour therapy for people with learning disabilities. Routledge, London, p 124–140

Masi G, Marcheschi M, Pfanner P 1997 Paroxetine in depressed adolescents with intellectual disability: an open label study. Journal of Intellectual Disability Research 41(3): 268–272

McGorry P 2000 The scope for preventive strategies in early psychosis: logic, evidence and momentum. In: Birchwood M, Fowler D, Jackson C (eds) Early intervention in psychosis. Wiley, Chichester, p 3–27

Mental Health Act 1983 HMSO, London

Neal M, Briggs M 2003 Validation therapy for dementia (Cochrane Review). In: The Cochrane Library, Issue 2. Update Software, Oxford

Nezu C, Nezu A, Arean P 1991 Assertiveness and problem-solving training for mildly retarded persons with dual diagnoses. Research in Developmental Disabilities 12: 371–386

Oliver P, Piachaud J, Regan A et al 2003 Difficulties developing evidence-based approaches in learning disabilities. Evidence-Based Mental Health 6: 37–39

Prout H, Cale R 1994 Individual counseling approaches. In: Strohmenr D, Prout H (eds) Counseling and psychotherapy with persons with mental retardation and borderline intelligence. CPPC, Vermont, p 103–142

Reiss S, Aman M 1998 Psychotropic medication and developmental disabilities: the international consensus handbook. Brookes, Baltimore

Reynolds F 1999 Creative arts, activities and therapies. In: Swain S, French S (eds) Therapy and learning difficulties. Advocacy, participation and partnership. Butterworth-Heinemann, Oxford, p 312–326

Rogers C 1961 On becoming a person. Constable, London

Rose J, West C, Clifford D 2000 Group interventions for anger in people with intellectual disabilities. Research in Developmental Disabilities 21: 171–181

Ruedrich S, Alamir S 1999 Electroconvulsive therapy for persons with developmental disability: review, case report and recommendations. Mental Health Aspects of Developmental Disabilities 2(3): 83–91

Ruedrich S, Noyers-Hurley A, Sovner R 2001 Treatment of mood disorders in mentally retarded persons. In: Došen A, Day K (eds) Treating mental illness and behavior disorders in children and adults with mental retardation. American Psychiatric Press, Washington, p 201–226

Rush A, Frances A (eds) 2000 Treatment of psychiatric and behavioral problems in mental retardation. American Journal on Mental Retardation 105(3): 159–226

Sainsbury Centre for Mental Health 2001 The capable practitioner. Sainsbury Centre, London

Sinason V 1992 Mental handicap and the human condition: new approaches from the Tavistock. Free Association Books, London

Sovner R, Fox C, Lowry M et al 1993 Fluoxetine treatment of depression and associated self-injury in two adults with mental retardation. Journal of Intellectual Disability Research 37: 301–311

Stenfert Kroese B 1997 Cognitive–behaviour therapy for people with learning disabilities: conceptual and contextual issues. In: Stenfert Kroese B, Dagnan D, Loumidis K (eds) Cognitive–behaviour therapy for people with learning disabilities. Routledge, London, p 1–15

Symington N 1981 The psychotherapy of a subnormal patient. British Journal of Medical Psychology 54: 187–199

Taylor D, McConnell D, McConnell H et al 2001 The Maudsley prescribing guidelines, 6th edn. Martin Dunitz, London

Tschudin V 1995 Counselling skills for nurses, 5th edn. Baillière Tindall, London

Tyrer S 2001 Psychopharmacological approaches. In: Došen A, Day K (eds) Treating mental illness and behavior disorders in children and adults with mental retardation. American Psychiatric Press, Washington, p 45–68

Van Meijel B, van der Gaag M, Kahn R et al 2002 The practice of early recognition and early intervention to prevent psychotic relapse in patients with schizophrenia: an exploratory study. Part 1 and Part 2. Journal of Psychiatric and Mental Health Nursing 9: 347–355; 357–363

Vaughan C, Leff J 1976 The measurement of expressed emotion in the families of psychiatric patients. British Journal of Social and Clinical Psychology 15: 157–165

Williams H, Clarke R, Bouras N et al 2000 Use of the atypical antipsychotics olanzapine and risperidone in adults with intellectual disability. Journal of Intellectual Disability Research 44(2): 164–169

Wray J, Patton K 2003 Complementary therapies. In: Gates B (ed) Learning disabilities: towards inclusion. Churchill Livingstone, Edinburgh, p 393–412

8

Mental health promotion

INTRODUCTION

This chapter will consider the role of policy, and the carer's role within the policy framework, in promoting the mental health status of people with learning disabilities. The wider concepts of public health, illness prevention, and health education will be explored, within the context of relevant health promotion models, as will the concepts of empowerment and the service user perspective, in the promotion of positive mental health in people with learning disabilities. Case study material introduced in previous chapters will be used to explore the practical application of mental health promoting strategies. Although mental health promotion is important internationally, the specific strategies discussed in this chapter relate mainly to the UK health, education, and social care context.

HEALTH PROMOTION

Health promotion, meaning, literally, a movement towards health, is a relatively recent concept that encompasses several fields of study (Tudor 1996). Its aim is to enhance positive health and prevent ill health by strengthening individuals, communities, and organisations. Thus, the key groups of people who can contribute to promoting health are the government, individuals in the community, and professionals in the field of health, education, and social care.

According to Tannahill (1985), there are three important and overlapping elements that contribute to the broad concept of health promotion: *health protection* (also referred to as public health), *health education*, and *illness prevention*.

Health protection/public health

The concept of health protection relates to the regulations, policies, and practices aimed at the prevention of ill health (Tannahill 1985), and in this sense it can be seen primarily as the responsibility of government and large organisations. It considers all causes of ill health and its treatment, and seeks to tackle the underlying causes of ill health and health inequalities (Department of Health 2001a). Historically, public health focused upon sanitation, epidemiology, disease, and the identification of health risks. More recently it has broadened to encompass the social networks that impinge on a person's life, including psychosocial aspects of health, unemployment, poverty, housing, social isolation, crime, and substance misuse. Thus, it is an approach which sees health within its overall social and political context, and looks for solutions in wider social action, individual empowerment, and community development, as well as in clinical interventions (Department of Health 2001a). It aims to build the capacity of communities to promote positive health at the same time as preventing disease by working with those communities in order to assist them to improve their individual and collective health.

Health education

This is a means of enabling people to change their health behaviours and practices through informing them about the links between behaviour and health, and is primarily the responsibility of health, education, and social care professionals, in conjunction with individuals, groups, and communities. The aim of health education is to enable people to make informed choices and decisions about their health, which should result in a permanent change in behaviour, beliefs or lifestyle. However, people are always at liberty to reject or ignore information and advice, particularly if it suggests that they need to make major changes to their lifestyle or daily activities. As an example, the public is informed in a variety of ways that smoking is harmful to health. However, many people, while accepting the information, choose not to stop smoking because it is an activity that they enjoy, or one that they share with family and friends, or one that helps them to deal with stress. So there is always a delicate interaction between health education messages (which may be seen as prescriptive) and the individual's interpretation and evaluation of those messages. Furthermore, powerful health education messages that are designed to shock people into changing behaviour are often unsuccessful. For example, one of the early advertisements warning against the dangers of HIV and AIDS, which showed a person's name being chiselled into a tombstone, was generally thought to be unsuccessful because it was so far removed from most people's everyday experience that they could easily argue that 'it won't happen to me'.

Illness prevention

In conjunction with public health and health education, a third and important strand of health promotion is prevention of illness. Prevention literally means to keep something from happening, so illness prevention means reduction of risk of disease (Tannahill 1985). For many years prevention of illness has been described as having three elements: primary, secondary and tertiary (Caplan 1964).

- *Primary prevention* seeks to prevent the first occurrence of a disorder and so decrease the number of new cases occurring in the community. In the context of mental health, this might be achieved, for example, through mental health educational programmes.
- *Secondary prevention* seeks to lower the rate or duration of established cases of a disorder, and might be achieved, for example, through the provision of counselling services for people who have been bereaved.
- *Tertiary prevention* seeks to decrease the degree of disability associated with a particular disorder, and might, for example, be achieved through the treatment of enduring mental health problems.

However, as prevention can only really happen before the incidence of a problem, it may now be more useful to think of a spectrum of interventions ranging from prevention through treatment and into maintenance, particularly in relation to mental health.

MENTAL HEALTH PROMOTION

Mental health problems cause significant disability to sufferers, and rank third after respiratory disease and cardiovascular disease in terms of their frequency in the population (Üstün 1998). Common mental health problems such as depression compare with hypertension, diabetes, and back pain in accounting for the number of days lost from work (Üstün 1998). Indeed, mental health underpins physical health in that people's social and psychological circumstances can damage their physical health in the long term (Department of Health 2001a). For example, depression increases the risk of heart disease and is a risk factor for stroke; sustained stress increases susceptibility to viral infection and physical illness (Department of Health 2001a). Clearly, then, it is in everyone's interests to reduce the incidence and ill effects of mental health problems wherever possible, and to increase individuals' capacity for positive mental health. So how can this be achieved?

Background and policy

Although mental health problems are extremely common, they are also diagnosable with greater precision than ever before, often treatable, and in many cases, preventable (Costa e Silva 1998). Despite this, it is of some note that many contemporary health and health promotion textbooks do not specifically refer to mental health promotion. This may not be surprising when we realise that it was not until 1992, with the publication in the UK of *The Health of the Nation* (Department of Health 1992), that improving the mental health of the population was identified as a national priority. Targets were set with the aim of improving the health and social functioning of mentally ill people and reducing suicide rates. Health promotion was recognised within this strategy document as a major contribution to improving the nation's general health. People with learning disabilities and their needs in relation to mental health were not, however, specifically included within this strategy; neither were they excluded. This can be interpreted as positive acknowledgement that people with learning disabilities have the same needs in relation to mental health issues as the rest of the population, and should have access to the same services, the philosophy espoused within the *Valuing People* strategy (Department of Health 2001b). However, as we shall see in Chapter 9, people with learning disabilities face many challenges in accessing mainstream services, so they may have particular difficulties in accessing health promotion generally (Coyle & Northway 1999), and mental health promotion services specifically.

Subsequently, the 'Health of the Nation' strategy was criticised for its emphasis on illness rather than on health and, by focusing upon steps that individuals should take towards meeting the targets, for instigating a culture of blame. More recently, *Saving Lives: Our Healthier Nation* (Department of Health 1999a), in which mental health, and particularly severe mental illness, remained a designated area of national priority, aimed to reverse this by highlighting the notion of partnership. The focus shifted away from the responsibilities of individuals and towards the partnerships that could be forged between individuals, local communities, and the government. In this way, opportunities were created for an increased awareness of mental health promotion.

This message has been reinforced internationally by the World Health Organization (1999) in its 'Health 21' targets. Target 6 focuses on improving mental health such that, by the year 2020, people's psychosocial well-being should be improved, and more comprehensive services should be available to and accessible by people with mental health problems.

In the UK, the *National Service Framework for Mental Health* (Department of Health 1999b) was published as a strategy to improve quality and reduce unacceptable local variations in the delivery of adult mental health services. Within this framework, which identifies a set of national standards to be achieved in five areas, Standard One addresses mental health promotion. Specifically, it aims to 'ensure that health and social services promote mental health and reduce the discrimination and social exclusion associated with mental health problems' (Department of Health 1999b). Groups of people that may be socially excluded, such as victims of domestic violence, black and ethnic minorities, and the prison population, are specifically identified within Standard One as being at risk of mental health problems, but people with learning disabilities are not identified as being a particular 'at risk' group. Subsequently, the Department of Health (2001a) published *Making it Happen*, a guide to the implementation of Standard One of the National Service Framework for Mental Health.

Defining mental health

As we have seen in Chapters 1 and 2, mental health itself is difficult to define. It is not simply the absence of mental illness. According to the World Health Organization, it also concerns the mental and social well-being of the individual (Üstün 1998). An early description of mental health suggested that its elements were mastery of the environment, an adequate perception of reality, integration, positive regard, continued growth to self-actualisation, and autonomy (Jahoda 1958). Tudor (1996) suggests that mental health is an integrative, generic term that has emotional, cognitive, behavioural, physiological, spiritual, and sociopolitical dimensions. These dimensions include coping, tension and stress management, self-concept and identity, self-esteem, self-development, autonomy, change, and social support, and that all of these can be assessed using specific assessment tools. Mental health influences how individuals feel, think, interpret events, and respond to change. It affects ability to learn, communicate, conduct personal relationships, and cope with change. Furthermore, as we have seen, it has a strong influence on physical health (Department of Health 2001a).

Individuals often find mental health a difficult concept to explain. Respondents in a survey of families in the North West of England found it difficult to find appropriate terminology, and tended instead to focus on mental *ill* health (Rogers & Pilgrim 1997). Interestingly, while these people tended to see external social factors as mainly responsible for mental ill health, they took personal responsibility for dealing with them, and in this way for maintaining mental health.

Defining mental health promotion

Just as mental health and ill health are difficult to define, so too is the concept of mental health promotion. But just as everyone has mental health needs, so everyone needs mental health promotion. It is the very opposite type of strategy to crisis intervention, which seeks to address problems once they have happened. The Department of Health (2001a) defines mental health promotion as involving 'any action to enhance the mental well-being of individuals, families, organisations or communities'. It can take a range of meanings including *treatment* of mental illness, *preventing the occurrence* of mental illness, *increasing resistance* to stress, and *enhancing resilience* when stress occurs (Loeb et al 1998). It can bring about improved physical health, increased emotional resilience, greater social inclusion and participation, and higher productivity (Department of Health 2001a). Furthermore, it can contribute to reducing discrimination and increasing understanding of mental health issues.

Models of mental health promotion

Referring back to Tannahill's (1985) model of health promotion, Verrall (1990) has provided examples of mental health promotion in the three overlapping elements of health protection, health education, and illness prevention. An example of mental health protection might be funding for teachers to run relaxation classes; an example of mental health education might be promoting self-empowerment; and an example of mental illness prevention might be the provision of counselling services. Where the three elements overlap, we have mental health protective education, an example of which might be educating managers about the need to support employees with mental health problems.

Within the prevention element of the model, Gordon (1987) suggests an alternative approach to the standard focus on primary, secondary, and tertiary elements. He suggests that the prevention element can be subdivided instead into the three categories of universal, selective, and indicated strategies:

- *Universal strategies* are targeted at the general public or a specific population of people such as pregnant women
- *Selective strategies* are targeted at those at higher risk than the general population of developing mental health problems
- *Indicated strategies* are targeted at individuals who have early indications of mental health problems but which are not yet formally diagnosed (e.g. improving coping skills following life trauma).

An alternative model of mental health promotion, which is drawn upon in *Making it Happen* (Department of Health 2001a), is provided by McDonald & O'Hara (1998). They describe ten elements of mental health promotion, five of which promote and five of which undermine the achievement of mental health. Promoting factors, which need to be strengthened, are quality environments, self-esteem, emotional processing, self-management skills, and social participation. The undermining factors, which need to be reduced, are deprived environments, emotional abuse, emotional negligence, stress, and social exclusion.

There are many other models of relevance to mental health promotion, but essentially what they all have in common is the need to reduce risk factors and increase protective factors.

Risk factors for mental health problems

Although it is fairly easy to see the link between some physical illness such as respiratory problems and risk factors such as smoking, it is more difficult to draw such links between risk factors for mental ill health and mental ill health itself. However, the Department of Health (2001a) has identified a range of factors that are known to increase the risk of developing mental health problems. These include bereavement, family history of mental health problems, childhood neglect, violence, financial difficulties, unemployment, family breakdown, and long-term caring. In addition, gender has an impact, with women having an increased risk of depression, eating disorders, and self-harm, and men being at higher risk of suicide than women. As we saw in Chapter 2, people with learning disabilities may be particularly vulnerable to mental health problems, hence it is vital that we take every opportunity to increase protective factors as much as possible to try to counteract the existing position of disadvantage that many people with learning disabilities experience.

Protective factors for mental health

Given this range of risk factors, we may ask ourselves whether it is possible to prevent mental ill health, yet prevention strategies are likely to be more effective than dealing with the consequent disorders once they occur (Üstün 1998). There are two broad processes that have the potential to protect mental health: community participation and empowerment.

- *Community participation* includes having significant attachments with other individuals and the opportunity to talk things over with others, to have access to support networks, and participation in meaningful activities.
- *Empowerment* is a process of helping individuals to develop autonomy in decision making. Empowering factors include positive self-esteem, increasing awareness of risk factors, the opportunity to learn new skills (including coping skills) and exercise creativity, economic security, job control, physical activity, and relaxation.

An example of empowerment that is growing in popularity is the *recovery movement*. This movement was established in the USA and New Zealand, and is now active within the UK. Recovery can be described as a means of promoting self-help, understanding one's own experiences of mental health problems, developing skills and knowledge to help oneself, and finding hope. In a survey of almost a thousand people with mental health problems in the UK, more than half felt that they had recovered from or were coping with a mental health problem (Baker & Strong 2001). Respondents cited spending time talking to friends and family, together with help from services, as key factors in helping them to keep mentally well. The main ified were negative attitudes of the general public and low self

MENTAL HEALTH PROMOTION AND PEOPLE WITH LEARNING DISABILITIES

If we consider the range of protective and risk factors described above we can see that people with learning disabilities are already at a disadvantage and at increased risk of developing mental health problems when compared with the general population. Prenatal brain damage, birth injury, intellectual disability, and low intelligence are all, in themselves, risk factors for the development of mental health problems. As we have seen throughout this book, many other adverse factors are likely to have been experienced by people with learning disabilities. These include peer rejection, poor attachment to school, school failure, abuse, unemployment, socioeconomic disadvantage, physical disability, loss, discrimination, and exclusion. They may have deficits in knowledge, attitudes, and understanding in relation to mental health (Shaughnessy & Cruse 2001). Consequently their mental health needs may be inappropriately or inadequately assessed, and intervention is likely to be inadequate or inappropriate. As a result, service provision may be poor or non-existent (Shaugnessy & Cruse 2001).

Equally, protective factors for mental health – such as economic security and job control – are often denied to people with learning disabilities. In addition, there are many professional barriers that stand in the way of effective mental health promotion for people with learning disabilities. Primary care has a key role to play and is being actively strengthened by the UK government (Department of Health 2001a). However, despite the fact that people with learning disabilities have a greater need for mental health promotion than the general population, there is evidence to suggest that their health needs are not being met by primary care services, and that they have a poor uptake of health promotion in general practice (Coyle & Northway 1999, Kerr et al 1997, Wilson & Haire 1990).

The reasons for this are many and varied, and include professionals' deficits in knowledge, attitudes, understanding and communication skills, lack of appropriate identification and referral systems for mental health needs, lack of valid and reliable assessment tools and outcome measures, time constraints, ritualistic working practices, and diagnostic overshadowing (explained in Chapter 1 as the tendency to interpret observed changes in mood and behaviour as part of the learning disability rather than as a mental health problem). Furthermore, individuals need to know where and how to seek help, and be physically able to do so, factors which, as we are aware, are sometimes denied to people with learning disabilities, who are often reliant on other people to identify their need for specialist help and to help them obtain it. However, although it is well accepted that people with learning disabilities do consequently have unmet health needs, these are not significantly different from the general population (Nightingale et al 1998), and it is argued that improvements in access to health promotion generally will incidentally benefit those with learning disabilities.

OVERCOMING BARRIERS TO HEALTH PROMOTION FOR PEOPLE WITH LEARNING DISABILITIES

Despite identified barriers, much can be done to address the mental health promotion needs of people with learning disabilities. As we have seen, health promotion works at the community, organisational, and individual level, and clearly we are reliant on the government and service providers to address some of the barriers to mental health promotion for people with learning disabilities, such as the provision of schools education programmes and GP education programmes. However, there is much that organisations and individuals can do to promote mental health. The most effective measures are likely to be selective strategies, targeted at people with a greater risk than others, and indicated strategies, where there are indications of a mental health problem that has not yet been diagnosed. We can think of many instances where people with learning disabilities might benefit from such indicated strategies, such as following a major life change, bereavement, or home move.

The provision of appropriate information can play an important part in empowerment and control, as confirmed by the Department of Health (1998) in its *Information for Health* and by the NHS Executive in its *Mental Health Information Strategy* (2001). These documents show how the provision of appropriate and accessible information in relation to looking after our own and others' mental health needs, self-help techniques, and service information can reduce fear and misconceptions about mental health problems, and support mental health care delivery. Of course, not all people with learning disabilities can access written information, and alternative means of providing information may be needed. Pictures and resources such as *Feeling Poorly* (Dodd & Gathard 2001) and those available from organisations such as the advocacy group People First (2002) can assist in the process of information transfer.

Other strategies that have been successful in the general population and that are emphasised in the 'Making it Happen' guidance (Department of Health 2001a) are increasing physical activity and relaxation activities. These activities are relatively simple and inexpensive to promote. Other strategies suggested are early interventions and early signs monitoring, as outlined in Chapter 7.

Of course, in the spirit of *Nothing About Us Without Us* (Department of Health 2001c), the people who can say most about what will help to promote their mental health needs are people with learning disabilities themselves. Two examples illustrate this point.

Example 1

In a survey carried out by the Estia Centre (Hardy 2002), service users with learning disabilities were asked what could help prevent them from developing mental health problems, and what they wanted in relation to mental health promotion. They described preventive factors as being treated as adults, having friends including boyfriends and girlfriends, being independent, having a social life, and not being afraid to speak up for themselves. They wanted services to educate them about protective factors rather than simply vulnerability factors, and to be able to access mental health promotion groups and support groups. Furthermore, they wanted to see the ideas proposed in *Valuing People* (Department of Health 2001b) and *Making it Happen* (Department of Health 2001a) put into practice. These comments support McDonald & O'Hara's (1998) strengthening factors.

Example 2

In addressing one of these strengthening factors – self-esteem – a local strategy was implemented by one of the authors (MG) and a colleague for a group of clients who had been diagnosed with depression. Fennell (1999) defines self-esteem as the overall opinion we have of ourselves, how we judge or evaluate ourselves, and the value we attach to ourselves as people. A series of six 90-minute self-esteem-raising group sessions was facilitated for six clients with a mild learning disability, aged between 18 and 23. The groups were aimed at reversing the stages described by Fennell (1999) as the process of developing low self-esteem.

- Stage one is *experience*, such as early childhood experiences through which ideas about the self, such as being the 'odd one out' are formed.
- Stage two is the *bottom line*, where individuals make conclusions, assessments and judgements about themselves.
- Stage three is *rules for living*, which are coping strategies that will help the person through their life.
- Stage four is *trigger situations*, where the rules are broken by, for example, being rejected, or the prospect of failure.

Once the trigger stage is activated then the bottom line maintains low self-esteem. The person produces negative predictions which confirm the low self-esteem, which in turn produces self-critical thoughts, which leads to depression. The 'bottom line' is then reactivated, producing a cycle of low self-esteem.

In the group sessions, techniques such as role play, role reversal, and cards to stimulate discussion were used. Homework was set and monitored via diaries. The negative impact of labels and stigma were discussed, as were issues of accepting people and valuing them for what and who they are.

Broader objectives were identified to empower the participants to control the sessions, to allow them to gain ownership of issues that worried them, and to develop a supportive friendship network. These sessions were evaluated positively by all participants and valued as a small contribution to the promotion of their mental health.

Exercise

Taking each of the people introduced so far through the case studies in this book in turn, identify:

- any specific risk factors for mental health problems
- any mental health promoting factors that are already available to them
- any additional health promoting activities that might be suitable in each case.

Geoff, who was introduced in Chapter 1, has experienced some recent changes in his life, such as a home change and change of living companions and carers. However, he is able to participate in meaningful activities within the home, and clearly has some creative talents and interests. He may benefit from an increase in physical activities, which in turn might contribute to an improvement in his sleep pattern. He may welcome the opportunity to engage in previous interests such as structured art activities within the community, and the opportunity to go on holiday or excursions.

Jason, introduced in Chapter 2, has also experienced some loss and change in his life. His father is no longer in the family home, and Jason appears to be experiencing pressure at school and at work. Furthermore, there is some suggestion that he feels physically unwell, which may be contributing to his withdrawal from activities and social contacts. In his favour, he has considerable support from his mother and his school, and has up to now participated in community life through employment and social activities. He is also normally physically fit and active. He might benefit from a structured programme of study support through the stressful examination period, and liaison with his school is clearly important here. Once this stressful period is over, it will be important for Jason to be helped to resume his previous interests and activities, while at the same time being supported through the transition between education and employment. The UK Connexions organisation exists to facilitate transition to adult life for all young people (with and without a disability) and it will be important to liaise with an appropriate personal advisor, who will also be able to help Jason discuss any problems affecting his school and family life.

Jenny, introduced in Chapter 3, is vulnerable to mental health problems. She has, in the short term, lost close contact with her family, has a limited degree of control in her life, and a very limited range of meaningful activities. These factors are compounded by the fact that she has poor verbal communication skills, and she also self-harms. She could benefit from an increased range of activities (including physical activities), from increasing her range of Makaton signs, and from an increase in self-esteem, perhaps by involving her in personal care activities such as a manicure, which might also distract her from her self-harming activities. Guided relaxation or massage sessions might also promote her general sense of well-being and reduce anxiety.

David, introduced in Chapter 5, has also experienced changes in his life through change of home owners and care managers. He has no verbal skills and has a physical disability. Furthermore, there appear to be some tensions with his parents. In his favour, he participates in the community through attendance at a college; however, his experience there is likely to be limited to contact with other people with learning disabilities. While his eye-rubbing behaviour might be a manifestation of some specific learning disability syndrome, and therefore difficult to eliminate, it might nonetheless be helpful to encourage David to participate in activities involving his hands, or requiring hand–eye coordination, such as board games, craftwork, or ball games, his physical disability permitting.

There is some evidence that self-harm may be an expression of depression in people with learning disabilities (Marston et al 1997, Sovner et al 1993), so a thorough screening for this for both David and Jenny is indicated.

These are suggestions only, and we do not wish to be prescriptive in suggesting appropriate interventions. You will, no doubt, by drawing upon your own experience of clients with specific needs and problems, be able to think of many additional mental health promoting strategies that would benefit these clients, and you may like to repeat the activity in relation to the case studies of Gordon and Ashia who will be introduced in Chapters 9 and 10, respectively.

CONCLUSION

As we have seen, mental health promotion is everybody's business. In the present political climate we are fortunate that government policy is actively promoting health promotion generally, and mental health promotion specifically, and is providing us with access to examples of good practice that might be adapted and implemented for people with learning disabilities. However, until such time as strategies to promote the mental health of people with learning disabilities are more specifically developed, local organisations, individuals, families and carers can make important inroads in some of the ways described, to the ultimate benefit of all people with learning disabilities.

In Chapter 9 we begin to explore the related issue of appropriate service provision for people with learning disabilities within the context of the legal, policy, and guidance framework.

REFERENCES

Baker S, Strong S 2001 Roads to recovery. Mind (National Association for Mental Health), London
Caplan G 1964 Principles of preventive psychiatry. Basic Books, New York
Costa e Silva J A 1998 World Health Organization perspectives and prevention of mental illness and mental health promotion in primary care. In: Jenkins R, Üstün T (eds) Preventing mental illness. Mental health promotion in primary care. Wiley, Chichester, p 7–12
Coyle D, Northway R 1999 Promoting health: the challenge for the community learning disability nurse. Mental Health Care 2(7): 232–235
Department of Health 1992 The health of the nation. A strategy for health in England. HMSO, London
Department of Health 1998 Information for health. An information strategy for the modern NHS 1998–2005. Department of Health, London
Department of Health 1999a Saving lives: our healthier nation. Department of Health, London
Department of Health 1999b National service framework for mental health: modern standards and service models. Department of Health, London
Department of Health 2001a Making it happen. A guide to delivering mental health promotion. Department of Health, London
Department of Health 2001b Valuing people. A new strategy for learning disability for the 21st century. Department of Health, London
Department of Health 2001c Nothing about us without us. Report of the Service Users Advisory Group in relation to 'Valuing People'. Department of Health, London
Dodd K, Gathard J 2001 Feeling poorly. Pavilion, Brighton
Fennell M 1999 Overcoming low self esteem. Robinson, London
Gordon R S 1987 An operational classification of disease prevention. In: Steinberg J, Silverman M (eds) Preventing mental disorders. A research perspective. National Institute for Mental Health, Rockville, MD, p 20–26
Hardy S 2002 Paper presented at the Mental Health in Learning Disabilities Special Interest Group Forum, Bradford University, 20 June 2002
Jahoda M 1958 Current concepts of positive mental health. Basic Books, New York
Kerr M, Dunstan F, Thapar A 1997 Attitudes of general practitioners to people with learning disabilities. British Journal of General Practice 46: 92–94
Loeb D, Markham W, Naidoo J et al 1998 Mental health promotion. In: Naidoo J, Wills J (eds) Practising health promotion. Dilemmas and challenges. Baillière Tindall, London, p 255–276
Marston G, Perry D, Roy A 1997 Manifestations of depression in people with intellectual disability. Journal of Intellectual Disability Research 41(6): 476–480
McDonald G, O'Hara K 1998 Ten elements of mental health, its promotion and demotion: implications for practice. Society of Health Education and Health Promotion Specialists, Glasgow
NHS Executive 2001 Mental health information strategy. NHSE, Leeds
Nightingale J, Ditchfield H, Pepperrel P et al 1998 Meeting the mental health needs of people with learning disabilities: a comparative study. Mental Health Care 2(2): 60–62
People First 2002 Access 2 pictures: a voice for people with learning disabilities. People First, London
Rogers A, Pilgrim D 1997 The contribution of lay knowledge to the understanding and promotion of mental health. Journal of Mental Health 6(1): 23–35
Shaughnessy P, Cruse S 2001 Health promotion with people who have a learning disability. In: Thomson J, Pickering S (eds) Meeting the health needs of people who have a learning disability. Baillière Tindall, London, p 126–157
Sovner R, Fox C, Lowry M et al 1993 Fluoxetine treatment of depression and associated self-injury in two adults with mental retardation. Journal of Intellectual Disability Research 37(3): 301–311
Tannahill A 1985 What is health promotion? Health Education Journal 44: 167–168
Tudor K 1996 Mental health promotion. Paradigms and practice. Routledge, London

Üstün T B 1998 The primary care setting – relevance, advantages, challenges. In: Jenkins R, Üstün T (eds) Preventing mental illness. Mental health promotion in primary care. Wiley, Chichester, p 71–80

Verrall J 1990 Mental health promotion – a framework. Cited in Tudor K 1996 Mental health promotion. Paradigms and practice. Routledge, London, p 61

Wilson D, Haire A 1990 Health care screening for people with mental handicap living in the community. British Medical Journal 301: 1379–1381

World Health Organization Regional Office for Europe 1999 Health 21: health for all in the 21st century. WHO, Copenhagen

9

Policy issues and service provision

(with contributions from Peter Bates)

INTRODUCTION

What should by now be very clear is that significant numbers of people with learning disabilities are likely to experience mental health problems at some time in their life, for which they and their families will require accurate assessment, diagnosis, treatment, and care. It follows then that there needs to be a robust system of service provision to ensure that these needs are met in a focused, targeted, and timely manner.

UK legal, policy, organisational, and practice frameworks endorse this need for appropriate service provision. There are a number of policies and guidance documents that specifically address mental health needs in people with learning disabilities such as *Count Us In* (Foundation for People with Learning Disabilities 2002) and *Psychiatric Services for Children and Adolescents with Learning Disabilities* (Royal College of Psychiatrists 1998). However, in the spirit of inclusion promoted by the *Valuing People* strategy for England (Department of Health 2001a) and *Improvement, Expansion and Reform – Ensuring That All Means All* (Valuing People Support Team 2002), the needs of people with learning disabilities should be included in all relevant policies that guide service development.

This chapter begins by giving an overview of some of the policies and professional guidance that should underpin good practice in service delivery. Perspectives from the Royal College of Psychiatrists, the Department of Health, and the voluntary sector will be discussed. Anti-discriminatory and anti-oppressive practice, equal opportunity, and access to mental health services for people with learning disabilities are themes that run throughout the chapter. Finally, the impact of the care environment will be discussed in relation to generic versus specialist service provision. The chapter provides illustrative case study material that will demonstrate the relationship between policy and effective care.

While examples from outside the UK are included, the bulk of the material within this chapter is set within a UK policy and service provision framework, and in some cases is restricted to the situation in England. This merely reflects the authors' country of origin, practice, teaching, and research, and should not be taken to exclude good practice in other areas.

THE UK POLICY FRAMEWORK

An effective service can only be successful if it is founded on nationally agreed policies. Any modern and comprehensive mental health service for people with learning disabilities and mental health needs should have its roots in mainstream or generic services (Hassiotis et al 2000), but we should also recognise that specialist services play an important role, not only in providing care for these clients but also in educating mainstream providers and family carers. By 'mainstream' or 'generic' services we mean those mental health services provided for the whole population, and by 'specialist' services we mean those services which provide knowledge, skills, and expertise to supplement mainstream services where needs cannot be fully met within those generic services. Specialist service provision varies widely across different parts of the UK, but examples might include assessment and treatment units, dually trained community nurses, consultant psychiatrists specialising in learning disabilities, or local psychological services.

The 1990s saw the emergence of several reports that identified the need for services for people with learning disabilities and mental health needs. In a book such as this it is impossible to consider all policies that influence service delivery, and therefore what follows is a brief description of some of the most relevant.

'Meeting the Mental Health Needs of People with Learning Disabilities'

This report by the Royal College of Psychiatrists (1996) was intended for psychiatrists providing services for people with learning disabilities and mental health problems. However, the main themes in the key recommendations are applicable to all professional groups working in this field. The four key recommendations are as follows:

- There is a need for specialisation to achieve high standards in services (including adherence to the legal and policy context, responsiveness to the views of carers and patients, and other factors to improve outcome).
- Comprehensive coverage requires attention to potential gaps in service provision (e.g. in relation to age, geography, diverse clinical needs, and patterns of service).

- Specialist multi-disciplinary mental health teams for people with learning disabilities and mental health problems are required to enable their clients to use ordinary health services wherever possible, and to provide help to meet the needs which cannot be met through the ordinary range of services.
- Joint working between specialists in the psychiatry of learning disabilities and other specialists should be promoted. A task for specialists is to improve the ability of other, less specialised services to serve people with mild learning disabilities.

What can be seen from this report is that services need to specialise in order to meet the needs of this client group, while at the same time making existing mainstream services accessible to people with learning disabilities. This report was followed in 1998 by a report that specifically examined psychiatric services for children and adolescents (Royal College of Psychiatrists 1998), which echoed this view, but which also stressed that in order for clients to access mainstream services, collaboration is imperative. Collaborative working should enable multi-professional networks so that families are not faced with negotiating a maze of services. In other words, clients and families should be able to access and benefit from mainstream services where appropriate, in the spirit of inclusion and anti-discriminatory practice, but should also be able to access speciality services to fill the gaps that mainstream services cannot fill.

'Valuing People'

For many years, Mencap, a UK charity that works for people with learning disabilities and their carers, had been concerned about the way in which services were provided for people with learning disabilities. There are many problems, including a lack of services and variations in service provision depending on where people live. People with learning disabilities are often not involved in making decisions about the services they receive. In 1999, the UK government commissioned research that confirmed this. Its report committed the government to developing a new national learning disabilities strategy for England, and work began on *Valuing People* (Department of Health 2001a) soon after this. The government formed six working groups, which included people with learning disabilities and carers, to look at the most important issues for people with learning disabilities and their families. The six working groups were:

- Health
- Supporting independence
- Children
- Family carers

- Workforce planning and training
- Building partnerships.

Mencap also reported to the government on what it wanted from a national strategy for people with learning disabilities. The summary of this report can be read in *New Targets for a New Century* (Mencap 2000).

There was also an advisory group of people with learning disabilities. They explained to the government what people with learning disabilities wanted their lives to be like and how they want services to work; their views are presented in *Nothing About Us Without Us* (Department of Health 2001b).

March 2001 finally saw the publication of *Valuing People* (Department of Health 2001a), a dynamic and forward-thinking White Paper. It outlines how people with learning disabilities should be cared for and who will be responsible for delivering that care. The Paper has four foci: rights, independence, choice, and inclusion.

Since the launch of *Valuing People* there have been many debates concerning its effectiveness and practical application, and since publication we are beginning to see the positive effects throughout service delivery systems. There are two driving forces – partnership and collaborative working, and person-centred planning – which will ensure that the four foci mentioned above remain at the forefront of all service and care developments.

Partnership and collaborative working

The concept of inter-agency working is not new. However, within *Valuing People*, the government set as a clear objective the need:

... to promote holistic services for people with learning disabilities through effective partnership working between all relevant local agencies in the commissioning and delivery of services.

(Department of Health 2001a, p 106)

One of the major vehicles for achieving this aim was to introduce partnership boards. Partnership is also not a new idea; many policies such as the Health and Social Care Act (2001) have included partnership as a core component. Partnership boards are responsible for local service delivery in the context of overall national policy. We have seen above how the Royal College of Psychiatrists advocated for collaborative working – but what is 'partnership', and how does this benefit people with learning disabilities and mental health problems?

Partnerships and collaborative working can only evolve if those involved share common ideas and philosophies. In the past, the development of isolated services has demonstrated that organisations sometimes have different ideologies. Unfortunately some services cannot (or do not) endeavour to meet the needs of people with learning disabilities and mental health problems. Some services have in the past discriminated against people with learning disabilities by denying them the skills and knowledge provided by the service. This discrimination is not necessarily intentional but rather a by-product of narrowly focused service development philosophies. The main aim of partnership boards is to achieve socially inclusive lives for people with learning disabilities, which are based on person-centred planning.

Partnerships work at three levels: strategic, operational, and individual.

- Agencies need to work together at a *strategic level* in order to share resources, for example through Health Improvement and Modernisation Plans (HIMPs). HIMPs are plans developed by local health authorities working in partnership with statutory, public, private, and voluntary organisations in order to improve health and modernise health services for local people by directing money, staff and services where they are most needed.
- At the *operational level*, it is expected that policies will drive service development, as illustrated, for example, by *Signposts for Success* (Department of Health 1998), which identified the core features of good quality health services for people with learning disabilities, and *Building Bridges* (Department of Health 1996), which guided service providers towards more effective inter-agency collaborative working. More recently we have National Service Frameworks that focus attention on partnerships, and these are discussed later in this chapter.
- However, it is at the *individual level* where these strategic and operational developments meet the person with needs. It is here that partnerships meet clients, listen to their views, and shape service provision to meet their needs in relation to access to services, staff training, and sharing information across agencies. All levels must ensure anti-discriminatory practice, and the production of policies and services must reflect this.

So, how can partnerships and collaborative working help someone who has learning disabilities and a mental health problem? Access to the appropriate service has often been problematic, with different organisational structures, local policies, and funding all impinging on the service provided. However, there are many examples throughout the UK where good services exist, for example see Singh et al (1994), Tyrone et al (1998) and Alexander et al (2001).

As with all service providers, there is constant emphasis upon providing the best quality service with the optimum use of resources, including funding. *Integrated care pathways* can help service providers to produce protocols based on locally defined, evidence-based, patient-centred best practice, in line with government initiatives. In essence, an integrated care pathway is a multi-disciplinary approach to care and service provision that aims to have the right people doing the right things in the right order at the right time in the right place with the right outcome, with attention focused on the client experience throughout. There are a range of elements that make up a care pathway, including:

- multi-agency activity
- evidence-based, locally agreed best practice
- local and national standards
- tracking facilities
- full documentation
- measurement of clinical effectiveness
- outcomes.

A care pathway can be seen as a definitive document that describes the process that will deliver care to the client and record any variation between planned care and the actual care delivered. It is a systematic tool that, by measuring against set standards, ensures consistent person-centred best practice, continuous improvement in patient care, and continuous feedback within a multi-agency context that incorporates agreed policies and guidelines. Ahmad et al (2002) have demonstrated how care pathways can be used with people who have learning disabilities and complex, chronic health problems. However, at the present time there are a limited number of care pathways in use for people with both learning disabilities and mental health problems.

Person-centred planning

The second driving force behind *Valuing People* is person-centred planning. Again, this is not a new concept within the field of learning disabilities, but it is worth considering in the light of associated mental health problems. Person-centred planning is a process in which service providers listen to each client and focus on what is important to that individual. From this the service should learn about the client's needs and wishes from the client's perspective. The fundamentals of listening and learning are the driving forces used as a basis to solve problems and negotiate the necessary resources to pursue the person's aspirations. Amongst other things, person-centred planning helps to direct and shape the contributions made from services, and thus clients become empowered.

There are five key principles that underpin person-centred planning:

1. The person is central to all aspects of their life, and person-centred planning is founded firmly on rights, independence, and choice.
2. Family members, other carers and friends are full partners in the planning of care.
3. Person-centred planning reflects the person's capabilities and what is important to that person, and specifies the support each individual requires to make a valued contribution to the community.

4. Person-centred planning builds upon a shared commitment that will uphold the individual's rights.
5. Person-centred planning leads to continual listening, learning and action.

We can thus see that people with learning disabilities can, with the help of others, take control of their lives and lead the way in fulfilling their needs, but what about the person who also has a mental health problem? This question may be more difficult to answer. As stated earlier, person-centred planning is a process, and there is a range of tools that can facilitate this process, common examples being Essential Life Style Planning (Smull et al 2001), Planning Alternative Tomorrows with Hope (PATH) (Pearpoint et al 1993), and Personal Futures Planning (Mount 2000).

In mental health services the philosophy of person-centred planning is encapsulated within *care coordination* (Department of Health 1999a), which updated both the Care Programme Approach (CPA) (Department of Health 1991) and the Social Services Care Management process. Care coordination is intended to reduce the duplication of documentation and confusion for clients, giving one assessment, one package of documentation, and one person to oversee the whole process. All people who are assessed as needing support from specialist mental health services will receive care under care coordination. The client – and where appropriate, their carer – is central to the whole process.

Care is delivered at two levels:

- *standard level*, where, by agreement between the client and the professional carer, the client's needs can be met with minimum support
- *enhanced level*, which is intended for more complex needs that require the support of a range of professional carers; this level facilitates communication between all involved.

At both levels clients can expect that their health and social care needs are assessed, that they are given a copy of their care plan, that a named person will coordinate the care plan and act as a contact point for all those involved in the care plan, that they will receive regular reviews, and be consulted throughout the care process. In theory, at least, people with learning disabilities who also have mental health problems should be able to access and benefit from the provisions of care coordination.

NATIONAL SERVICE FRAMEWORKS

In the late 1990s the UK government began a programme of national standard setting (National Service Frameworks, NSF), in order to raise quality and reduce variance in the provision of health and social services. Standards were set in relation to a wide range of health conditions such as coronary heart disease, diabetes, and mental health, and to specific age groups such as children and older people. As we saw in Chapter 8, the *National Service Framework for Mental Health* (Department of Health 1999b), in developing the government's mental health strategy *Modernising Mental Health Services: Safe, Sound and Supportive* (Department of Health 1999c), focuses on the mental health needs of all working age adults. Although they are not specifically mentioned within the NSF, people with learning disabilities of working age are implicitly included within the framework. The NSF applies to both health and social service provision, and includes health promotion, assessment, diagnosis, treatment, rehabilitation and care, including support to carers, and encompasses primary and specialist care and the roles of partner agencies. The framework sets national standards and defines service models for promoting mental health and treating mental illness.

The National Service Framework for Mental Health has seven standards. As we saw in Chapter 8, *Standard One* concerns health promotion. Specifically, health and social services should:

... promote mental health for all, working with individuals and communities, and combat discrimination against individuals and groups with mental health problems, and promote their social inclusion.

History informs us that people with learning disabilities have often been excluded from society. This standard may go some way to reducing the exclusion experienced.

Standard Two states that:

Any service user who contacts their primary health care team with a common mental health problem should have their mental health needs assessed and be offered effective treatments, including referral to specialist services for further assessment, treatment and care if they require it.

Standard Three continues this theme of access to services by stating that any individual with a common mental health problem should be able to make contact around the clock with local services. Arguably, people with learning disabilities and mental health problems are likely to experience problems in accessing services. This chapter highlights some of the difficulties that can result in discrimination towards people with learning disabilities seeking access to mental health services. Although it has been shown that people with learning disabilities do experience all common mental health conditions, these are often manifested in ways different from those seen within the general population, and it may be that only a small number of mental health service staff are aware of this. Thus there could be problems when creating 24-hour services for this population.

Standard Four indicates that all mental health service users on the CPA (now care coordination) should 'receive care which optimises engagement, prevents or anticipates crisis, and reduces risk'; they should have a copy of the correct documentation, and be able to access services 24 hours a day, 365 days a year. Anecdotal evidence suggests that people with learning disabilities are now using care coordination successfully to facilitate access to mental health services, although there is little research evidence to substantiate this view.

Standard Five states that:

Each service user who is assessed as requiring a period of care away from their home should have timely access to appropriate placements which is in the least restrictive environment, being cognisant of their needs. This placement should be as close as possible to their home. On discharge, a written copy of the care plan should set out the care and rehabilitation to be provided which identifies the care coordinator and specific actions that need to be taken.

As this chapter will identify, not all mainstream services have the facilities, expertise or knowledge to cater for people with learning disabilities with mental health needs, and providing access to services close to home may currently be difficult. There are some services, such as 'dual diagnosis units' or 'assessment and treatment units', that are within the geographical location of mainstream mental health services, but these tend not to be managed by the service. In relation to copies of care plans, not all people with learning disabilities can read, so there is no guarantee that they will be able to understand what has been planned for their future.

Standard Six relates to the carers who provide regular care for a person on the CPA (now care coordination), and states that these carers should have access to assessment of their own needs on a regular basis, and have their own copy of the CPA (now care coordination). The effects on families of caring for a person with learning disabilities and mental health problems will be discussed further in Chapter 10.

Finally, *Standard Seven* states that local health and social care authorities should prevent suicide by:

- promoting mental health
- delivering primary mental health care
- providing access to relevant services, including 24-hour services
- providing care plans that meet the needs of individuals with severe and enduring mental health problems.

They should provide safe hospital accommodation for those who need it and provide the support that people with severe mental illness need to receive to continue their care.

In considering the impact of the NSF for mental health we must be cognisant of the fact that although people with learning disabilities are not specifically identified as an at-risk group for mental health problems, under the inclusive philosophy of 'all means all', people with learning disabilities and mental health problems can and should benefit from the provisions of the NSF.

Perspectives from the voluntary sector: the example of the Judith Trust

In the UK there exists a range of services that could be helpful to people with learning disabilities, and their families, who may have mental health needs. It is not just the NHS and social services departments that provide services, care, skills and knowledge for people with learning disabilities and mental health problems. There are also several voluntary organisations, for example the Judith Trust. The Trust is a charitable organisation focusing specifically on people with learning disabilities and mental health needs. The Trust aims to improve the quality of life of people with both learning disabilities and mental health problems, and to support multi-disciplinary approaches to care delivery. The Trust commissioned a report that reviewed current services and projects (Kurtz 1999), which highlighted many examples of good practice, but also identified issues of concern, including the many barriers to providing good services to meet the mental health needs of people with learning disabilities. The case study of Gordon illustrates some of the difficulties in accessing appropriate services.

Case study: Gordon

Gordon, 36, has mild learning disabilities and lives at home with his parents. His father is a self-employed builder and often takes Gordon to work with him. Gordon also attends a social service day centre 2 days a week. His mother works part-time in the local corner shop on the same days that Gordon attends the day centre. Gordon appears to be a confident person and has good communication skills. He likes to be the centre of attention and often plays jokes on people at the day centre.

Staff at the day centre have noticed that over the last 6–12 months his behaviour has changed. He has become over-confident, loud and demanding. He tells people that he owns a large national building company and that is why he only attends the centre twice a week. When questioned about this he explains in great detail the latest projects in which his company is involved. For example, he explains how he built the 'London Eye', and how he had to have many meetings with his accountants because at one stage he thought that he might go bankrupt.

At home Gordon behaves as though he is his father's employer and that his mother is his secretary. He makes constant demands of his parents, who do what they can to meet these demands. Gordon sincerely believes that he is the head of a large building company. He offers to take people to buildings where he and his father have worked and explains that they have built these buildings. In reality they have done minor repair works inside the buildings.

Recently Gordon demanded that his father block the back door of the house with high quality building materials so that his accountants could not get in. When his father refused, Gordon 'sacked' him, telling him to leave the house and not return. He is becoming extremely disruptive both at the day centre and at home, and his father is now losing business because of Gordon's presence in the workplace.

The community nurse feels that Gordon may have a mental health problem, and has referred him to the psychiatrist. To ease the pressure on the family, the community nurse has also referred Gordon to the local assessment and treatment unit, a specialist service that aims to help people with learning disabilities and mental health problems or challenging behaviours, but there is a waiting list and there is no other suitable service locally that can meet his needs. His mother is suffering from stress but is refusing to let Gordon go to a social service respite hostel.

Gordon appears to have some signs of psychotic disorder. He appears to have delusional ideas, some of which are grandiose in nature (e.g. believing that he owns a large building company) and some of which appear persecutory (e.g. he appears to be afraid of the accountant). However, it must not be assumed that these are delusional ideas without further investigation. We must clarify whether what appear to be false beliefs are in fact misunderstandings or misinterpretations due to his level of intellectual functioning. As stated earlier in this book, the quality of psychotic symptoms in people with learning disabilities can be different from those of the general population. As we have seen, in the general population a person suffering from delusions holds their beliefs very strongly; however, in people with learning disabilities it is sometimes possible to 'talk them out' of their false belief (Royal College of Psychiatrists 2001). This is important to bear in mind when interviewing clients during assessments.

At the start of interventions with Gordon, his needs should be considered in conjunction with those of his family. Gordon and his parents have specific, immediate needs. For Gordon, he needs an initial assessment made by the appropriate professional. A screening tool such as the PAS-ADD Checklist or Mini PAS-ADD (see Ch. 6) could initially be used, which would at least give some indication of specific areas of mental health functioning in which there might be problems. This could be completed in conjunction with his parents and the staff at the day centre. At this stage Gordon may not be willing to participate in direct assessment. His parents are likely to need some form of support for their immediate needs. They may benefit from counselling, respite care, or education that informs them of Gordon's problems and how to begin dealing with his delusional ideas and behaviour.

In terms of service provision, it is tempting to imagine a range of services that would perfectly address both Gordon's and his family's immediate and long-term needs. However, service provision often falls short of perfection. There are, though, certain key elements that should be considered when attempting to create an effective service for people with learning disabilities who also have mental health needs. As a result of a literature review and informal survey of service providers in the UK and elsewhere, carried out by one of the chapter authors (PB), seven key elements were identified. These are summarised in Box 9.1 and are discussed subsequently.

Box 9.1   Elements of an effective service

- Overall strategy
- Collaboration
- Service planning and finance
- Research, evaluation and audit
- Staff skills
- User involvement
- Access to services

An overall strategy for people with learning disabilities and mental health needs

It is important to develop an overall strategy. The Mental Health Act Commission 7th Biennial Report (1997) notes that local agreements for the provision of services for patients with mental health problems and learning disabilities are urgently needed. Rubinstein (2000) found that the absence of effective joint planning, commissioning, and providing services for people with dual needs contributed to the death of Lorna Thomas. Lorna Thomas had mild learning disabilities and mental health problems and was admitted to a mental health care centre where she met and developed a relationship with a fellow voluntary patient. They were discharged within 6 days of each other. One month later Lorna Thomas was found with severe injuries in the home of her friend and died the same night. Her friend was convicted of her murder.

Any service that provides care for people with either learning disabilities or mental health problems should have an overall strategy for how people who have dual needs will be served. The strategy should be based upon inter-agency collaboration, along with effective joint planning and funding. Each stakeholder should share the same common values and service goals. A good strategy should:

- lead to focused planning, common assessment, service access points, dissemination of best practice, and joint staff training
- facilitate the provision of community-based support, 24-hour crisis response, institutional and community treatment programmes, the capacity for day and housing programmes, case management, family support, and specialised services to respond to people with learning disabilities and mental health problems
- be accessible to all relevant people including service users and their carers. A team should monitor the implementation of the strategy, quickly identify problems and resolve them. The strategy should involve an action plan.

Collaboration

Within the UK there are many examples of good practice that contain the above elements, such as pooling health and social service budgets and encouraging community mental health teams and community learning disabilities teams to work collaboratively. Although some services have managed to achieve such collaboration there are many difficulties.

1. Many mental health and learning disabilities services are underfunded, thus leading to inadequate provision. In this case, joint working will be sacrificed, or be seen as relevant to only a small number of service users, and so the process may fall into disuse.
2. Managers often lack experience of working across both learning disabilities and mental health services, and this leads to hesitancy in assembling a coherent and robust strategy. Effective collaboration can be helped by staff who have a commitment to bringing learning disabilities services and mental health services together for the benefit of people with dual needs, but it can soon be eroded by individuals who have no such commitment.
3. There is a problem that we might call 'arguing over the head of the user'. If a learning disabilities organisation has neglected to develop a strategy for collaboration with their mental health colleagues, sooner or later a person will come along who clearly requires the expertise of both services. Care planning for the person is then caught up in 'arguing over the head of the user'. Instead of focusing on the needs of the person, staff may feel that an offer to assist this client will set a precedent. Inevitably, the ensuing discussions about the principles delay the provision of a proper service to the person, and may cause it to be withheld entirely.
4. Some services have written strategies but they are couched in very general terms in order to allow for local interpretation. The danger here is that they can be so imprecise that practitioners ignore them.

Collaboration is a consistent theme throughout services; however the structures required to facilitate good collaboration are often complex. In this section we examine in detail the collaboration that is needed between staff working in learning disabilities services and their colleagues in mental health.

There are a number of recent factors that have increased the difficulty in establishing and maintaining good working relationships between learning disabilities and mental health staff. Social services take the lead on care for people with learning disabilities, while health services take the lead on mental health. Even within a single agency, the tasks of commissioning learning disability services and mental health services may be undertaken by different people.

The increased number of NHS trust formations and mergers is dislocating informal relationships between mental health and learning disabilities services and putting mental health services in different trusts from their learning disabilities colleagues. As a result, staff do not see each other so often.

Whilst there has been a growth in the partnership between social services and health, these arrangements could have been at the expense of collaboration between learning disabilities and mental health services. Government initiatives such as the development of partnership boards, care pathways and joint investment plans have brought people together, but this has only rarely included people from mental health services joining together with colleagues from learning disabilities services.

The different attitudes and cultures within the two services can be combined with an aversion to shared care to produce an approach that uses eligibility criteria to exclude anyone who does not neatly fit.

Finally, some mental health service areas are not co-terminous with their learning disabilities counterparts and this automatically creates a barrier to collaboration.

These barriers are being tackled by some agencies; one inner city Learning Disabilities Partnership Board, for example, is bringing together both health and social services under a single management system. Here a city-wide mental health service for adults with learning disabilities has been agreed to enable the requirements of the National Service Framework for Mental Health to be met for people with learning disabilities. The details are set out in a service specification.

In order for effective services to develop at field level, both mental health and learning disabilities teams should communicate with each other, share ideas, skills and knowledge, and be centrally managed. The setting up of a liaison person is useful to forge links. Establishing protocols and service agreements can enhance collaboration; for example, in parts of the UK there are agreements between the community teams 'never to refuse' to do a joint assessment; the teams meet for joint training on a regular basis and the practice of shadowing each other is supported. Some teams agree protocols on pre-admission, on ward care, and post-discharge arrangements. Other areas have team members who specialise in mental health issues in people with learning disabilities, and these specialists can be based either within the learning disabilities team or within the mental health team. There is an exchange of knowledge, skills, and clinical expertise.

Throughout the UK there are examples of collaborative initiatives. For example, in one area in the north of England, people from the learning disabilities service now participate in a 'diversion panel' and a 'multi-risk panel' alongside mental health, police, and probation colleagues. Here they jointly consider the needs of people who are in danger of entering the criminal justice system or those who are presenting serious risk behaviours, and develop shared approaches and plans (Cole 2002).

Other examples of service developments include specialist teams consisting of psychologists and school nurses working together, specialist interest groups, and newsletters. Transitional plans for young people moving from child to adult services have been developed between neighbouring trusts and authorities. In some low security units, learning disability and mental health nurses work together.

Shared care is in its infancy but the concept has real potential as two different agencies with differing philosophies can share responsibility for the planning and administration of a client's care package.

Service planning and finance

Services should be planned in response to the needs of the people who live in the area. However, in Chapter 1 we saw that there are difficulties in relation to research methodology, classification systems, and diagnostic tools that have to be overcome by anyone seeking to identify how many people with learning disabilities have mental health needs. As a result, any attempt to record the numbers of people with overlapping needs is likely to be flawed.

Poor data about the number of clients with mental health needs make it very difficult for policy makers and service providers to identify sources of funding and other resources that would enable them to provide effective services. A further barrier to an effective service is created when one service makes changes to their system without reviewing the implications for the other service. Change that could be of great benefit to both services is marred when staff have difficulties in thinking beyond the boundaries of their own service.

However, in some parts of the UK attempts are being made to ensure that clients are identified and then receive the appropriate service. Examples include:

- The development of transitional services which assist people through key stages of their life.
- The use of specific assessment tools such as PAS-ADD (Moss et al 1996) and HoNOS-LD (Roy et al 2002) (see Ch. 6) to identify people, especially those with mild learning disabilities.
- Writing eligibility criteria that relate to the treatment of mental health problems in people with learning disabilities rather than just the recognition of it.
- Identifying the people that 'don't fit' into neatly designed services and those that meet several eligibility criteria, as required by *Fair Access to Care Services* (Department of Health 2002). This may bring to light some clients who have gone unnoticed for many years or people who have been receiving the wrong treatment.
- Making a commitment to a seamless service in order to lower the barrier between learning disabilities and mental health services. Joint working parties across learning disabilities and mental health services aimed at addressing issues of common concern are developing in the UK. This approach develops better policies and fosters good communication.

- Holding regular joint meetings where 'difficult to allocate' referrals can be discussed and care can be planned, monitored and audited.

Coherent service development is sometimes impeded by the differences in financial charges between health and social services that interfere with the creation of care packages. In addition to the fact that health care is free at the point of use, while social care clients can be charged, commissioners may find themselves influenced by different charging arrangements for various services. For example, accommodation and care in a continuing health care bed is entirely chargeable to health, while the same person might be supported in their own home and be able to claim welfare benefits for the care component. This indicates that commissioners need to be fully aware of the cost of specialist services for the mental health needs of people with learning disabilities, as well as the cost of repeated psychiatric hospitalisation and admission to assessment and treatment units.

Where clients require support from a range of services, a multi-agency perspective needs to be taken in calculating costs. A carefully planned programme should include the costs required to provide an effective service without wasteful expense. In the USA the 'DOORS model' (Smith 1999) is a system developed by the State of Wyoming that facilitates the decision making process in order to match funding, services and the client's needs. The system identifies a flexible 'individual resource allocation' (IRA) that allocates a sum of money to individuals rather than to services. When care teams, including the client and their family, plan care packages they are aware of the funding. The DOORS model measures 60 factors including IQ and secondary diagnoses in order to calculate an individual budget for each person's care. This model has been in operation for over 12 years and shows a cost reduction over time.

Research, evaluation and audit

An effective service must be firmly based on research evidence, and local continuous evaluation is required to ensure high quality service provision. Until recently, there have been no national audit services that relate specifically to the mental health needs of people with learning disabilities. However, the Foundation for People with Learning Disabilities published a report in 2002 relating to young people with learning disabilities and mental health needs which is discussed further in Chapter 10. Throughout the UK there are local initiatives to review services. Care pathways are being developed that will contribute to service evaluation.

Staffing issues

As staff interpret and deliver the policies and protocols of their services, one of the central components of an effective service is the knowledge and skills of the staff. As an example, nursing has, within the UK, traditionally had four discrete branches: adult, child, mental health, and learning disabilities. The mental health and learning disabilities branches are of most relevance to people with learning disabilities and mental health problems yet each one tends to exclude the other. Indeed, it has been suggested that nurses in both these fields deliver primarily *physical* nursing care, and although this is an important component of holistic care delivery, nurses are capable of providing a much broader range of services (Cutler 2001). Cutler provides some recent evidence from the USA that suggests that mental health nurses are becoming more involved in assessment, treatment, patient advocacy, consultation, and education of staff and families of people with learning disabilities and mental health problems.

Many health trusts in the UK have offered additional training to registered nurses in the learning disabilities RN(LD) field so that they are able to gain the registered nurse (mental health) qualification. However, it appears that many of these dually trained nurses are still unable to synthesise their learning and straddle the gap between learning disabilities and mental health in terms of knowledge, skill, assessment, and intervention (Gibbs & Priest 1999). Indeed many retrained staff have subsequently gone on to work in the mental health field rather than returning to implement their new knowledge and skills within learning disability services.

A range of resources is available to support in-service training for staff. These include 1 day events and training packs. Some agencies provide mandatory updates while others encourage people to seek advice by arranging drop-in advice services for carers or staff. There are also a limited number of post-registration courses devoted to the education and training of RN(LD) nurses in the mental health needs of people with learning disabilities, including some at diploma and degree level. The courses that are available have been evaluated positively, and these programmes appear to be much more successful in helping nurses to integrate their learning and bridge the gap between mental health and learning disabilities services than is possible by gaining separate qualifications in both fields.

The evaluation conducted by Gibbs & Priest (1999) of one such course showed that the participants were able to develop their perceptions of the client group, which aided service delivery. Throughout the UK there are examples of similar short in-house courses that help to meet local needs. Despite these initiatives, it is disappointing to find that the mental health needs of people with learning disabilities tend to be an optional extra rather than an essential component of care. While a few areas in the UK are investing heavily in mental health training and education for their community learning disabilities teams, others adopt a different stance. Some believe that people with learning disabilities and mental health problems should access mainstream mental health services and therefore do not provide specialist mental health training and education to their learning disabilities services. Other agencies have a high proportion of unqualified staff with minimal training and may not even provide services for clients with mental health problems.

Current government policy advocates collaborative working. However, unless there is close working over a period of time, staff may simply attend case reviews and give reports without ever gaining a sense of the perspective or values of staff from the other agency. Currently there does not appear to be any formal way in which staff are educated about each others' roles. Attempts to introduce other agencies during nurse education programmes are generally confined to information about formal responsibilities rather than the roles, philosophies, and skills that could benefit clients with a mental health problem.

User involvement

As part of Gordon's care we can expect that his carers would attempt to involve him in his care planning. Though this is sometimes difficult, carers should encourage Gordon to participate. Despite the fact that user involvement is no longer a new concept, and we can see examples of clients organising and participating in conferences, undertaking advocacy roles, and campaigning for better services, there is no national service user group for people with learning disabilities and mental health problems. People with learning disabilities and mental health problems are not often heard about in the academic literature or on conference platforms. In an effective service, user involvement must be paramount. This can be achieved in a variety of ways, including:

- the use of information leaflets that are designed to be accessible to people with learning disabilities
- interviewing clients to find out about their needs and satisfaction with services
- training for clients who sit on partnership boards or other such committees and organisations
- training for advocates, carers and other user supporters. This would increase the number of learning disabilities advocates with knowledge of mental health issues, and the number of mental health advocates with knowledge of learning disabilities.

For a service to meet the needs of people with learning disabilities and mental health problems, the service planners must find out about the choices people have, how they express and communicate those choices, what obstacles there are to clients making those choices, and what things support people and help them to understand what is going on in their life. By doing this the service will facilitate the user having more input and control in their mental health treatment and in the ways in which services are run.

Access to services

Access to appropriate services is one of the biggest barriers that Gordon and other people like him will face. After identifying his needs and goals the nurse should be able to ensure that appropriately skilled staff are available and accessible to address these needs. Sometimes a bed in a hospital or other in-patient facility such as a mental health resource centre is needed.

Unfortunately it is often difficult to access a bed in an in-patient facility, so people with learning disabilities and mental health problems who need admission to hospital tend to go out of the area to neighbouring trusts that specialise in learning disabilities. This fails to achieve the goal of locally based services as advocated by the government (Department of Health 2001a). Mental health service beds are often used only when all assessment and treatment unit beds are full, and clients are returned to the assessment and treatment unit as soon as a bed becomes available there.

People with learning disabilities often receive a poor level of care in mental health units (Mental Health Act Commission 1997). They often need a longer stay on psychiatric wards, which makes them appear 'difficult' for busy wards used to a high throughput. High staff turnover can be a feature of psychiatric admission wards and this can cause concern for clients with learning disabilities who stay longer, see staff changes, and take longer to form relationships. Some people with learning disabilities need practical help with self-care, such as help to wash, dress, eat, and use toilets, which may not be readily available in busy acute mental health facilities. Finally, people with learning disabilities may not receive the right services. The Mental Health Act Commission (1997) notes that patients who lack capacity are rarely sectioned under the Mental Health Act; they are often described as having challenging behaviour and, as we have noted in previous chapters, are often treated with continuous and high doses of medication.

Children with learning disabilities and mental health problems also need access to the appropriate service. The development of mental health services for children with learning disabilities has lagged behind that for non-learning disabled children with mental health needs (Bernard 1999).

In order to resolve some of these access difficulties, there should be an agreed protocol for access to services and a commitment from managers to working in partnership. This would lead to some or all of the following practical outcomes:

- Clients who receive mainstream psychiatric hospital care should receive care from psychiatrists who have sufficient skills and knowledge in learning disabilities psychiatry.
- The in-patient facility to which the client is admitted should have access to registered nurses (learning disability) at all times. This may mean that one or more team members on every shift is a qualified RN(LD).

Services beyond the acute in-patient facility also matter:

- In a crisis response team there must be staff who are skilled and knowledgeable in the mental health needs of people with learning disabilities.
- Outreach services should be responsive to people with learning disabilities and mental health needs.
- All services should be non-discriminatory and allow any person who can benefit from their service access to the range of skills and knowledge provided by its staff. In the English Midlands there are examples of drop-in services for people with mental health problems, including those with learning disabilities.

History tells us that service providers can never get it right. The 1950s and 1960s saw institutional care at its peak with some 70 000 residents in England and Wales living in such places. In Chapter 1 we reviewed the history of learning disabilities care and noted how services have swung backwards and forwards between community and institutional care. The White Paper *Better Services for the Mentally Handicapped* (DHSS 1971) began to focus service providers' thoughts on what was required by people with learning disabilities, and stimulated service planning for the future needs of people with learning disabilities. It recommended that people should live in the community, in 'small' 200-bedded units. However, the White Paper did make a stand for community care and will be a useful source of guidance for many years to come.

Generic versus specialist service provision

As we have indicated throughout this chapter, the question of whether people with learning disabilities and mental health problems should access mainstream generic mental health services that meet the needs of the population as a whole, or whether there should be specialist service provision, remains largely unanswered.

The roots of the generic services argument can be found in the philosophy of normalisation, which advocates that all people with learning disabilities should be exposed to the culturally normative experiences of the society in which they live; this includes receiving generic services as available to the general population. There is considerable support for the view, however, that provision within ordinary mental health services, whether by default or design, cannot satisfactorily meet the total needs of people with learning disabilities and mental health or behavioural problems (Day 1995).

Day (1995) provides evidence from both the USA and Europe which confirms that generic service provision alone is unsuccessful. Poor staff training, lack of skills and knowledge, and lack of time and resources are cited as some of the reasons why generic services are not totally effective for this client group, whereas within specialist services, care staff from within learning disabilities are likely to be more knowledgeable about learning disabilities and about therapeutic interventions that work with these clients. This book has demonstrated how an awareness of mental health needs can lead to appropriate assessment and diagnosis with the aid of appropriately designed and selected tools, and to the provision of therapeutic intervention adapted to suit the clients' needs. Care staff are becoming aware that mental health problems can manifest in different ways, and that people with learning disabilities sometimes express fears of other services. Specialist services can bring together the skills and expertise of professional carers.

On the other hand, there are some disadvantages of specialist services; for example, specialist services go against the philosophy of community integration and inclusion. It may be, too, that generic services meet the needs of some clients with some problems, while specialist services may be appropriate for other clients with different problems. Alexander et al (2001) compared two major models of in-patient services for people with learning disabilities and mental health problems, namely the specialised assessment and treatment service model and the mainstream mental health service model. Preliminary findings suggest that there were some differences in the profiles of the clients that each model attracted; the specialist unit model attracted more people with severe disabilities and those with pervasive disorders compared with the mainstream service model. It is likely, then, for the foreseeable future that as 'one size does not very often fit all', both approaches to service delivery for this client group will be required.

CONCLUSION

The UK government has stated clearly that people with learning disabilities and mental health needs should access mainstream psychiatric services wherever possible (Department of Health 2001a). These services will become more responsive and be supported by specialist help from practitioners from the learning disabilities field. The government has also indicated that the National Service Framework for Mental Health is applicable to people with learning disabilities of working age, and that it supports a seamless service (Department of Health 2001a). The government will take steps to enable people with learning disabilities and mental health problems to access the services that meet their individual needs, by ensuring that:

- mental health promotion material is produced in an accessible format for people with learning disabilities
- strategies for improving services such as housing and education will be cognisant of mental health well-being
- protocols will be established that lead to collaboration between local mental health and learning disabilities services

- close collaboration between services will ensure that care is delivered via health action plans, and that care coordinators have experience in both mental health and learning disabilities fields
- specialist staff from learning disabilities will be available to provide support where necessary in time of crisis
- each local service will provide acute assessment and treatment services for people with learning disabilities who cannot access mainstream psychiatric services.

What can be seen from this chapter is that the concept of a perfect, needs-led service is an elusive one. However, service providers and policy makers are making a commitment to people with learning disabilities and their carers to provide a substantial service that is inclusive, based in mainstream services but supported by specialist services as appropriate.

REFERENCES

Ahmad F, Bissaker S, de Luc K et al 2002 Partnership for developing quality care pathway initiatives for people with learning disabilities. Part l: Development. Journal of Integrated Care Pathways 6: 9–12

Alexander R T, Piachaud J, Singh I 2001 Two districts, two models: in-patient care in the psychiatry of learning disabilities. British Journal of Developmental Disabilities 47(2): 105–110

Bernard S H 1999 Mental health services for children and adolescents with learning disabilities. Tizard Learning Disabilities Review 4(2): 43–46

Cole A 2002 Include us too: developing and improving services to meet the mental health needs of people with learning disabilities. King's College Community Care Development Centre/The Judith Trust, London

Cutler L A 2001 Mental health services for persons with mental retardation: role of the advanced practice psychiatric nurse. Issues in Mental Health Nursing 22: 607–620

Day K 1995 Psychiatric services in mental retardation: generic or specialised provision? In: Bouras N (ed) Mental health in mental retardation: recent advances and practices. Cambridge University Press, Cambridge, p 275–292

Department of Health 1991 The care programme approach for people with a mental illness referred to specialist psychiatric services. HC(90)23/LASSL(90)11. Department of Health, London

Department of Health 1996 The health of the nation: building bridges. Department of Health, London

Department of Health 1998 Signposts for success. Department of Health, London

Department of Health 1999a Effective care coordination in mental health services: modernising the care programme approach: a policy booklet. Department of Health, London

Department of Health 1999b A National Service Framework for mental health: modern standards and service models. Department of Health, London

Department of Health 1999c Modernising mental health services: safe, sound and supportive. Department of Health, London

Department of Health 2001a Valuing people: a new strategy for learning disabilities for the 21st century. Department of Health, London

Department of Health 2001b Nothing about us without us. Department of Health, London

Department of Health 2002 Fair access to care services: guidance on eligibility criteria for adult social care. Department of Health, London

DHSS 1971 Better services for the mentally handicapped. HMSO, London

Foundation for People with Learning Disabilities 2002 Count us in: the report of the committee of inquiry into meeting the mental health needs of young people with learning disabilities. The Mental Health Foundation, London

Gibbs M, Priest H M 1999 Designing and implementing a 'dual diagnosis' module: a review of the literature and some preliminary findings. Nurse Education Today 19: 357–363

Hassiotis A, Barron P, O'Hara J 2000 Mental health services for people with learning disabilities. British Medical Journal 321: 583–584

Health and Social Care Act 2001 The Stationery Office, London

Kurtz Z 1999 Joined up care: good practice in services for people with learning disabilities and mental health needs. The Judith Trust, London

Mencap 2000 New targets for a new century: learning disability strategy. Mencap, London

Mental Health Act Commission 1997 Seventh Biennial Report. The Stationery Office, London

Moss S, Goldberg D, Patel P et al 1996 The psychiatric assessment schedule for adults with a developmental disability: PAS-ADD. Hester Adrian Research Centre, Manchester

Mount B 2000 Personal futures planning: finding directions for change using personal futures planning. A sourcebook of values, ideals, and methods to encourage person centred development. Capacity Works, New York

Pearpoint J, O'Brien J, Forest M 1993 PATH: a workbook for planning positive possible futures. Inclusion Press, Toronto

Roy A, Matthews H, Clifford P et al 2002 The Health of the Nation Outcome Scales for people with learning disabilities (HoNOS-LD). Royal College of Psychiatrists, London

Royal College of Psychiatrists 1996 Meeting the mental health needs of people with learning disabilities. Royal College of Psychiatrists, London

Royal College of Psychiatrists 1998 Psychiatric services for children and adolescents with learning disabilities. Council Report CR70. Royal College of Psychiatrists, London

Royal College of Psychiatrists 2001 DC-LD (Diagnostic criteria for psychiatric disorders for use with adults with learning disabilities/mental retardation). Gaskell, London

Rubinstein V 2000 Report of the independent inquiry into the care and treatment of Lorna Thomas and Nicolas Arnold. Buckinghamshire Health Authority, Amersham

Singh I, Khalid M I, Dickinson M J 1994 Psychiatric admission services for people with learning disabilities. Psychiatric Bulletin 18: 151–152

Smith G 1999 Wyoming DOORS: setting individual resource allocations for HCB services. National Association of State Directors of Developmental Disabilities Services, Alexandria, VA

Smull M, Sanderson H, Allen B 2001 Essential life planning – a handbook for facilitators. North West Training Development Team, Manchester

Tyrone T, Treadwell L, Bhaumik S 1998 Acute in-patient treatment for people with learning disabilities and mental health problems in a specialised admission unit. British Journal of Developmental Disabilities 44: 20–29

Valuing People Support Team 2002 Improvement, expansion and reform – ensuring that all means all: handy hints for primary care trusts and strategic health authorities. Department of Health, London

10

The family and carers' perspective

INTRODUCTION

One of the largest groups of carers is the family. There are many estimates of how many family carers exist. The Princess Royal Trust (1998) gives a figure of six million carers in the UK and the government acknowledges that families provide the bulk of support for people with learning disabilities (Department of Health 2001a). Indeed, it is estimated that around 60% of adults with learning disabilities live at home with their families (Emerson et al 2001). This final chapter draws attention to the family and the everyday realities and challenges presented by individuals with complex needs, from the perspective of clients, their families and other carers. It will explore the effects of having a family member with learning disabilities and a family member with mental health problems. Due to the fact that the concept of mental health problems in people with learning disabilities has only gained prominence in recent years there is limited literature available in relation to the families of such people, and in particular about the effects of this dual disability upon the family members. However, much is known about family stress where there is a member with learning disabilities; equally there is considerable evidence relating to the effects on the family where a member has a mental health problem. It can be surmised therefore that where both problems coexist, stress within the family will be considerable.

To help determine whether this supposition is correct, and to go some way towards filling the deficit in the literature, the authors have spent time with families who have a member with learning disabilities and a mental health problem, and will call upon these experiences to illustrate family concerns and reactions. The chapter begins with an overview of the effects of learning disabilities and mental health problems on the family, and then explores a range of issues that impact on the family when both problems coexist. With reference to a case study, the concepts of social inclusion/exclusion, life transitions, and emotions will be explored. The chapter predominantly considers children and young people within the context of the family, but also pays some attention to the needs of older carers.

FAMILY STRESS IN LEARNING DISABILITIES

In this section we will explore some of the research from the past two decades that demonstrates how having a child with learning disabilities can affect the mental health of the parents, and particularly the mother. Wyngaarden-Krauss (1994) defines parental stress as 'dimensions of parental functioning (for example depression, sense of competence, and relations with spouse)'. Although families of children with learning disabilities report more stress than families of children without learning disabilities (Beckman 1983, Friedrich & Friedrich 1981), there is considerable diversity in the way in which this stress is expressed. Stress can be seen as a response to events or changes that alter an individual's social setting. This response may consist of one or more physiological or psychological reactions that can be both immediate and delayed. Thus a number of events, such as financial difficulties, marital problems, depression, and isolation, amongst others, have been considered indicators of high levels of stress.

Friedrich & Friedrich (1981) designed a study to determine whether parents of children with learning disabilities differed from parents of children without learning disabilities in terms of the variables of stress and also the variables that can relieve stress. Findings supported their hypothesis that significant differences would exist, with families of children with learning disabilities experiencing more stress and less marital satisfaction, psychological well-being, social support, and religiosity. Friedrich & Friedrich (1981) suggest that these significant differences are important as parents of infants, preschool children, and adolescents may face more intense stress during initial adjustment to the child's disability or when the child reaches puberty.

Wilton & Renaut (1986) compared 42 mothers of intellectually impaired preschool children with 42 mothers of non-intellectually impaired preschool children, to ascertain whether or not stress levels were different. Results showed that mothers of children with learning disabilities experienced higher levels of stress. Fathers were not included in the stress measures, suggesting that fathers were perceived as not being at risk of stress or not having a major role to play in the family.

Breslau & Davis (1986) reported on the effects of chronic stress of mothers of children with disabilities. Their primary question was: 'Do persons who differ with respect to the stressfulness of their life situation show different risks for major depression?' Specifically they compared mothers of children with congenital disabilities with mothers of children free of disability. Mothers were asked to rate symptoms such as mood, loneliness, loss of appetite, sleep disturbances, and concentration problems. The results showed that the mothers of the children with disabilities had more depressive symptoms when compared with the control group.

In a further study, Ryde-Brandt (1990) assessed anxiety and depression in 18 mothers whose children were diagnosed as having learning disabilities and autism or other pervasive childhood psychosis and who were receiving some form of special education. The control group contained 18 mothers of physically handicapped children, none of whom had learning disabilities and all of whom attended mainstream schools. The mothers of children with autism scored significantly higher on the Hospital Anxiety and Depression (HAD) scale (Zigmond & Snaith 1983) than mothers of physically handicapped children.

In contrast to these findings, some studies have shown that stress is no more likely in families with a child with learning disabilities than in families without. Ryde-Brandt (1988), for example, examined the occurrence of anxiety and depression in 13 mothers of children with Down's syndrome aged 8–9 years, and compared them with 13 female supporting care assistants who were helping the mothers. The HAD scale (Zigmond & Snaith 1983) was used to assess the feelings of anxiety and depression, and a semi-structured interview was used to collect additional data. The scores for the mothers of children with Down's syndrome and for the supporting care assistants indicated that there was no evidence of depression or anxiety occurring in either group.

While these results are in contrast to Ryde-Brandt's later work (1990), this study's control group comprised paid care assistants rather than mothers. The difference is therefore perhaps unsurprising, as these carers would be unlikely to have had 24-hour responsibility for the children, and furthermore, would be unlikely to share the same degree of emotional attachment to the children as the mothers.

Bristol et al (1988) compared depressive symptoms in the mothers and fathers of 31 preschool boys with autism and other communication disorders with mothers and fathers of 25 non-disabled boys. They hypothesised that the parents of disabled boys would show higher levels of depressive symptoms. One of the specific goals of the study was to determine if adaptation varied with the gender of the parent and the disabled/non-disabled status of the child. Both groups were matched on child race, gender, and mean age as well as parental status, mean parental age and socioeconomic position. The results of the study show that although mean scores for depressive symptoms for both mothers and fathers of disabled boys were higher than those for the control group, the differences were not statistically significant.

Cameron et al (1991) found that parents of developmentally delayed children do not report stress in their family environment. The aim of their study was to measure the stress experienced by parents of developmentally delayed and non-developmentally delayed preschool children. The developmentally delayed children had a variety of conditions including Down's syndrome and cerebral palsy. The measure used was a 121 item self-report questionnaire with two dimensions:

1. *The child's characteristics* – a high score obtained on this scale indicates that the child displays qualities that might make it difficult for the parents to fulfil their parental role.
2. *The parental domain* – a high score in this domain indicates that stress may occur.

When the mothers of the developmentally delayed children were compared with the mothers of the non-developmentally delayed children there were no differences reported in depression, the degree of attachment to the child, the amount of restrictions on the parental role, the amount of social isolation for the mother, or the relation that the mothers had with their spouse. Cameron et al (1991) suggested that the mothers of developmentally delayed children had been able to make adjustments in their life and were able to deal with the problems raised by the child's handicapping condition.

Although several of these studies seem to indicate that parents of children with learning disabilities are no more likely than any other parents to experience stress, nonetheless it is difficult to draw definite conclusions because studies have used different populations, measured different variables, used different methods of collecting data, and used different measurement tools to draw their conclusions. It may be that having a child with learning disabilities does increase the risk for parents of developing a range of difficulties relating to stress, but whether or not stress is activated will depend on a wide range of personal and environmental factors, such as coping strategies and social support. We will explore these factors later in this chapter.

Family stress and mental health problems

As we have seen, and in common with changing philosophies in learning disability care, there has been a shift from institutional and hospital care of people with mental health problems to care in the community. This means that as people develop mental health problems, their treatment, accommodation, and general day-to-day care is more likely to occur within the family setting. Families of people with mental health problems often take on the role of primary caregiver, either voluntarily or by default. This applies even when the family member is receiving in-patient care. There are numerous studies that identify the negative effects on families, such as anger, embarrassment, shame, guilt, blame, and exhaustion. Families must quickly learn coping skills as well as ways of understanding and helping their relative. Yun-Hee & Madjar (1998) suggest that some families cope by living each day as it comes. They conclude that caring for a family member with chronic mental health problems is experienced both personally and in the fabric of family relationships. It is different from the role and experience of the professional carer who is essentially a stranger to the situation.

Much has been written about the effects of mental illness on the family. As we saw in Chapter 7, much of what is known focuses on family members with either schizophrenia or depression. Pejlert (2001), for example, studied the parents of six adult sons/daughters with schizophrenia over a period of time, and attempted to illustrate the meaning of parental caregiving, which emerged as a lifelong effort involving sadness, having difficulty in interpreting the symptoms of mental illness, and struggling to find out what was wrong. Once the diagnosis had been explained they then entered a bereavement process, just as parents of learning disabled children do when they discover their child's disability. At this stage, families in Pejlert's study reported emotions of shock, confusion, anger, guilt and despair, and grieving for the loss of the son or daughter they once had. Some parents were reminded of this by the presence of healthy siblings. Parents reported that they had accepted the mental illness but not the consequences, and those who had come to terms with their child's illness coped in many different ways. Some became actively involved in advocacy services, others in their child's care package, and others concentrated on thinking positively and having their own interests and activities.

The effects of having a child with schizophrenia can be seen within different cultures. Pejlert's study was conducted in Sweden where the adult children were receiving care in long-stay organisations and had regular contact with their families. However, in Hong Kong, Wong (2000) highlighted additional difficulties in a culture where family care is seen as imperative and where families take on the primary role and responsibility for caregiving, even when a family member has schizophrenia. Although as we have noted, many people in the UK similarly take on the primary caring role, what makes a difference in Hong Kong are the cultural issues such as 'face saving'. In the Chinese culture, the 'face' of the family represents the image and prestige of the family in public. Mental illness in Hong Kong remains highly stigmatised so many families who have a member with mental health problems try to save face and hide the shame that the person brings to the family. With cultural issues being accounted for, Wong's study showed that carers of people with schizophrenia experience difficulties and stress, particularly in relation to the negative symptoms, such as refusal to perform household duties and neglect of personal hygiene. However, they experience less stress in relation to the positive symptoms of schizophrenia such as bizarre communication and behaviours resulting from hallucinations and delusions (Wong 2000).

Clark & King (2003) have also identified that caring for a family member can have negative effects on the carer. In their study of caregivers of people with strokes and Alzheimer's disease, a large number had depression scores above the level indicating clinical depression even when services such as respite and support were provided.

In relation to the role of carers of people who have depression, Keitner & Miller (1990) reviewed a range of studies that identified adverse effects on family functioning, communication and problem solving. This was supported by Tamplin et al (1998) whose study showed that the general health of families of young people with major depression was significantly worse than in a control group. However, while the mothers' mental health was poor, the fathers' mental health state was not related to family functioning.

On a positive note, there is a range of research supporting the notion that if families are more involved in the caregiving and treatment of people with mental health problems then they are better equipped to deal with the stress of mental health problems in the family. For example, Whelton & Pawlick (1997) reported on a community rehabilitation programme in which families of people with schizophrenia were included in the rehabilitation team, and were provided in turn with support and educational programmes. With this level of support, families reported increased satisfaction and fewer worries about their caregiving role. Similarly, in relation to Alzheimer's disease, Marriott et al (2000) demonstrated how the involvement of the family in cognitive–behavioural interventions can actually improve the mental health of family caregivers.

The family and people with learning disabilities and mental health problems

We often think of caregiving as a negative concept but we should accept that it can also be a positive experience, producing a sense of satisfaction (Bulger et al 1993). Each family member is unique and thus the dynamics of each family will differ; the effects of learning disabilities and mental health problems will impact on each family in myriad ways. McIntyre et al (2002) suggested that expressions of mental health in learning disabilities can be expected to heighten family stress and influence parental decisions about services. They also demonstrated that mental health problems in learning disabilities affect maternal stress above and beyond the stress contributed from other young adult and family characteristics. Hence it is important for professional carers to be aware of the potential effects, to involve families in all aspects of care and intervention wherever possible, and to offer appropriate supports, as illustrated by the case study of Ashia.

In previous chapters we have discussed the importance of accurate assessment but have also identified many of the barriers faced when trying to assess mental health problems in people with learning disabilities. The

---

Case study: Ashia

Ashia is 18 years old with mild learning disabilities and epilepsy. Until recently she lived at home with her family, and attended a special needs unit at the local comprehensive school. Her mother stays at home and looks after Ashia's younger sisters, Varuni, 9, who attends the local primary school, and Shamila, 16, who is completing her final year at the same comprehensive school. Ashia's father is a project manager for a local engineering firm and is able to work from home several days a week. Both parents are active members of the local Mencap support group and have strong views on the rights of people with learning disabilities and their families. They often hold meetings in their home.

Ashia is now working in a small food preparation unit within a sheltered employment organisation. Her transition into the workplace was well managed by education and social services. Recently Ashia has moved into a flat with Natalie, a friend since childhood, who also has mild learning disabilities. The young women are supported by an independent living scheme, and a care worker from the scheme drops in every day. Natalie tends to rely on Ashia to run the flat, as she gets frustrated when dealing with money and doing jobs around the house. Recently the care worker has noticed that the flat is exceptionally clean and tidy, and often smells strongly of disinfectant. When approached about this Ashia becomes a little agitated and avoids the conversation, simply saying she's house-proud like her mum.

The independent living scheme carers are also concerned about changes in Ashia's behaviour: she has become quiet over the past 6 weeks, she sometimes does not take her medication for her epilepsy, and has been isolating herself in her room. For these reasons the team have referred her to the local community nursing team for an initial assessment.

Exercise

- What should the community nurse do first of all?
- What are the indications that Ashia may have a mental health problem?
- What anxieties might Ashia and her family have experienced in the period leading up to Ashia moving away from home?
- How might the family remain involved in Ashia's life now that she has left home?
- How might the professional carer help the family to adapt to Ashia's move?

---

initial response of the professional carer should be to arrange to meet with Ashia, attempt to develop a therapeutic relationship, and take a detailed history in order to discover why her behaviour and mood might have changed. Formal assessment tools may contribute to the process.

Care workers have identified a preoccupation with cleanliness. Is Ashia just being house-proud, or is this indicative of an obsessional problem? It might be that Ashia is missing the routine and familiar surroundings of her family and home, and is trying to create some sense of stability and order in her life.

Ashia's parents too may be worrying about how she is coping with the move. They may still be coming to terms with the 'loss' of their daughter and the fact that they are not always on hand to help and guide her. They may be experiencing loss of role as parents and carers of a person with learning disabilities, particularly parents who are actively involved in support groups, and may even feel rejected. They now have more time to spend with the other children in the household, and the dynamics of the family will change. The professional carer should aim to involve the family in Ashia's life and future by suggesting to her that her parents would be welcome to join in any planning meetings that will take place. As her parents are already involved with Mencap they could use this organisation as a source of support at this time.

The mental health needs of children and young people with learning disabilities

Today the family is recognised as central to the care process and is seen as a crucial aspect of service effectiveness (Department of Health 2001a). The concept of the family is diverse, and there are many definitions. Giddens (2001) notes that the 'traditional' nuclear family of two parents and two children has gradually been eroded, resulting in a greater diversity of family forms. Family forms are just as diverse where there are learning disabled members, with a multitude of relationships (Grant & Ramcharan 2001).

Let us now turn our attention to the younger members of the family. Unfortunately children are not immune to mental health problems and recent attention has been paid to the plight of these young people. The Foundation for People with Learning Disabilities (2002a, p 7) has stated that:

Young people with learning disabilities are at high risk of developing mental health problems – more so than young people who do not have learning disabilities.

In Chapter 1, we discussed the difficulties inherent in ascertaining the prevalence rates of mental health problems in people with learning disabilities. These same difficulties are just as relevant to children and young people with learning disabilities and mental health problems. What we do know is that in the age range 13–24 there are in the order of 8.7 million people who live in Great Britain. Of these, there could be in the region of 750 000 young people with learning disabilities (Foundation for People with Learning Disabilities 2002a). If the prevalence rates for mental health problems across all age groups are mirrored for children and young people, and are around 40% as suggested by Emerson (2003), then we could expect that up to 300 000 will have additional mental health problems requiring a specific service response.

How can young people with learning disabilities be protected from developing mental health problems? Firstly, as soon as a problem has been identified or diagnosed families can benefit from early intervention, and it is here that schools, nurseries, and play groups can be involved in developing partnerships with the family to assist the child through their early years. Understandably, there is a reluctance to label such young children as having mental health problems, as any difficulties may be temporary and due to developmental or social factors. However, mental health problems may become more noticeable, and demand more attention, as children approach teenage years. At this time they enter a key transitional period of their life which marks the growth from childhood to adulthood, and by the move from school to college or, hopefully, to meaningful employment.

Being a teenager can be a stressful time, when insecurities commonly revolve around what the future holds in relation to education, employment, and relationships. Some teenagers find it difficult to develop relationships, and have anxieties relating to sexuality, image, and identity. For young people with obvious outward signs of disability, they may begin to realise how their differentness can lead to stigma and bullying, which may in turn lead to low self-esteem, anxiety, and depression. Furthermore, as people with learning disabilities become teenagers there may be a realisation that they may not achieve their dreams and aspirations as older siblings may have done. Jo, for example, in one of the families we talked to, has an older brother who has just started college, and who intends to study mechanical engineering at university. Even though teachers and her family try to create a realistic picture and not build up her hopes, Jo finds it difficult to accept that she will never be able to attend university. The perceived lack of support to follow her dreams leads to low self-esteem, and eventually Jo's mood spirals downward into depression.

There is evidence to suggest that during the transitional period young people in the general population are at a high risk of developing mental health problems, and that this risk is even higher for people with learning disabilities (Masi 1998). The transition period has attracted much attention in recent years. Organisations are now providing services to support young people through their teenage years; however, our families reported that there is still little preparation for or information about the transfer from child to adult services. This view is widespread, and there is evidence to suggest that many young people with learning disabilities leave school without a transition plan, that they have little or no involvement in planning for their future, and that the quality of transition varies widely (Norah Fry Research Centre 2002).

Key issues for families

We have previously noted that there is as yet little literature pertaining to the needs of families of people with learning disabilities and mental health problems. In this section, therefore, we draw upon discussions held with families where one member had both learning disabilities and a mental health problem. The youngest 'client' in the families we spoke to was 15 and the eldest 62; all but one live at home with their parents, with the remaining person living in a small group home with four other people with similar abilities. In discussing these families, the identified client with learning disabilities is sometimes referred to, for convenience, as the 'child' within the family, even when this person is chronologically an adult. Discussions were focused around the following themes:

- 'Being told'
- Effects on the family of the disability/illness
- Emotions and relationships within the family
- Coping strategies
- Parent/family training
- Services
- Facing the future.

'Being told'

A significant factor in the lives of these families was the way in which they were told that their child had learning disabilities. Families need the supporting role of professional carers, from the first diagnosis to the development and instigation of successful treatment plans. Most of our families, in hindsight, felt that 'being told' had been carried out in an appropriate and supportive way, apart from the family of the 62-year-old who had been advised to find institutional care for their child, reflecting the social attitudes of the time. What was noticeable was the way in which families dealt with being told that their child had a mental health problem. This sometimes re-establishes the emotions that the family had experienced when they were first informed of the diagnosis of learning disabilities. When families are faced with the news of illness or disability they can react in a variety of ways; some families freeze as they cannot cope with the news and deny the need for support or services. It is here where, in the classic bereavement process, families stay at the denial stage. Alternatively, the family might accept the situation and develop coping skills to create an environment around them and their child that helps to support them. Carers have to use their communication and counselling skills to help the family to work through the new emotions and will have to be able to explain diagnostic criteria, assessment tools, and the terms and language used by other professionals.

Our families agreed that while they had come to terms with the fact that their child had learning disabilities, the news that they now had a mental health problem dealt most families a 'double blow', causing them to embark on a grieving process all over again. However, one family said that it was just another factor in their child's life that they [the family] would have to deal with.

Effects on the family of the disability/illness, and relationships with professional carers

Families have been recognised as the largest group of caregivers (Williams & Robinson 2001a), and most of the families we spoke to actually felt that they were the sole carers, responsible for the care of their child 24 hours a day. Ideally, professional carers and families should have an agreement about exactly who the client is (in other words, is it the identified 'client' or is it the whole family?) and where the duty of care lies; however, this does not always happen.

Barr (1996) has identified a range of models that explain the ways in which professionals work with families. These models range from the professional being classed as an expert, with the family simply obeying instructions and being passive recipients of wisdom and decisions; to the negotiating model where active participation on behalf of the family is encouraged and where the family has control over decisions. In such a model, both parties learn from each other. Our families reported experience with the first model; namely that professionals often took control of the situation and did not allow the family time to reflect and become empowered. Some families were left out of the assessment process even though they felt capable of contributing to such assessments. This could lead to the fragmentation of care, interventions not being fully understood or implemented, and a breakdown of the relationship between the family and professional carers.

Dale (1996) suggests that parental involvement is vital to the care process and suggests that professional carers need family cooperation in order to fulfil their role effectively. Family members are key resources in the implementation of assessments and interventions; however, they need support and guidance to help them carry out these responsibilities. We must also recognise that the clients themselves have their own needs and wishes which may not necessarily be the same as those of the family in which they live.

The partnership between families and professionals is as complex as the family itself, and the creation and development of such a relationship can often be a difficult and complex journey for both sides of the partnership (Grant & Whittell 2000). Both parties must recognise each other's role; the role of the professional carer is to facilitate the family's ability to maintain its function in order to support both itself and the member with learning disabilities and mental health problems. One of the functions of the professional carer is to discover the dynamics of the family, to be aware of who the client relates to and in what way, and be aware of the effects of professional input on other members such as siblings. The families we spoke to felt that they had a good relationship with professional carers and that these professional carers had a good understanding of the dynamics of the family.

Emotions and relationships within the family

As predicted by Williams & Robinson (2001a), some of our families had experienced relationship problems and conflict within the family, either between partners or with the client's siblings. They had developed their own strategies to deal with these problems, and only one family had sought professional help for relationship problems. Most families expressed concern for the siblings of the client; comments such as, 'they don't bring friends home' or 'they don't want to play with their brother because he always breaks their things' were common. Adult siblings were more concerned with who was going to care for the identified client when the parents are no longer able to do so. The majority of families commented on how supportive their own, sometimes elderly, parents were and that without them they could not cope. Grandparents were a good source of informal sitting services, counselling, respite and financial support.

Coping strategies

Families had developed a wide range of coping strategies to enable the family to function in as 'normal' a way as possible. For example, times when the child with learning disabilities was in respite care would be used to devote time to other children, and to do 'normal' things such as eat a meal together. Families had learnt to 'read' and interpret the client's mood and act accordingly. Their coping strategies varied according to the services that were available to them. Some were able to access respite services, but provision varied from area to area and was in some cases minimal. One family became involved with voluntary organisations and helped to run self-help groups as a way of dealing with the stress and emotional burden of caring. They were able to meet and talk through the problems and pleasures of having a child with learning disabilities and the new experiences of emotional difficulties.

These factors may be illustrative of the concept of resilience, whereby a family develops the ability to withstand and rebound from crisis and distress. Heiman (2002), in a study of 32 parents, identified three main factors that enabled parents to function in a resilient way:

- They need to be able to have open discussions with their family, their friends and professionals.
- There needs to be a positive bond between the parents which helps to support and strengthen them.
- There needs to be continuous educational, therapeutic, and psychological support for all the family.

All the families could identify individual professional carers who were very helpful in facilitating adjustment and coping; these included the family doctor, the community learning disabilities nurse, the special school, and the local social service day care centre staff. However, they could also identify gaps in service provision that they felt would be beneficial to their family member, and all families were able to tell stories of long waiting times, poor communication, and feeling let down. However, it is to their credit that none wished to complain about any service; indeed they were very appreciative of the services that they were receiving.

Parent and family education and training

Families will need information about the mental health problems experienced by their children in order to develop appropriate skills and interventions. This might be accessed through parent and sibling training. Van den Borne et al (1999), for example, reported that parents of children with Prader–Willi syndrome and Angelman syndrome had a high need for information relating to the future consequences for their child and how they might develop in the future; they also experienced high depressive feelings and feelings of loss of control. If a client has an identified mental health problem then the professional carer should be educating all members of the family and not just the immediate carers. Their understanding of the concept of mental health in learning disabilities will encourage them to participate in care delivery and may also encourage and deepen the personal relationships between family members.

Within the families we spoke to, few had been offered family education or training in how to deal with emotional expression or challenging behaviour, although this would have been welcomed.

Services

Young people with learning disabilities and mental health problems suffer the commonly identified mental health problems such as depression, schizophrenia, anxiety disorders, and obsessive–compulsive disorders. What is important is how carers and service providers attempt to provide the optimum care through appropriate screening, assessment, and diagnosis followed by an intervention programme individually tailored to meet the young person's overall health needs. When a family first think that there may be a problem with their child they should contact their GP and primary health care team who should be able to coordinate and guide the family through the supporting agencies.

It is not only the GP that should be able to help. Within the government's philosophy of inclusion, support for the family should come from a range of services. Education services within schools, educational psychologists, paediatricians, the Connexions service and school health services can intervene alongside specialist services from community learning disabilities teams, mental health service, and social services. Advocacy services will also be useful in helping families to find their way through the maze of services and ensure their rights are met.

Assessment and clear diagnosis is vital as it will drive the appropriate interventions. Families may be asked to participate in family therapy or other psychotherapeutic interventions, all of which may appear difficult or strange to the family and should be explained by the carer who has a detailed knowledge of such therapies. Families need to be informed of issues such as their legal rights, and issues of consent need to be addressed.

Plans need to be made to address the future of the family member who has learning disabilities. More complex problems need to be referred to appropriate services, and it is here that many families encounter problems. Services for young people, though developing, are not consistent across the country. At the macro level, 10 years ago the NHS, in a review of Child and Adolescent Mental Health Services (CAMHS), proposed a four-tier model of service delivery (Williams & Richardson 1995) which should ensure that the needs of all young people, regardless of the complexity of their needs, are met with the appropriate degree of support.

- *Tier One* services offer first-line services to the public from agencies such as GPs and health visitors.
- *Tier Two* interventions are provided by individual specialist mental health workers.
- *Tier Three* services are more specialised and are offered by teams.
- *Tier Four* services are highly specialised to respond to very complex cases such as in-patient and secure provision.

Though service philosophies have developed in the last 10 years, the principles of the four-tier model are still current today.

More specifically at the micro level, when a family has a child with learning disabilities, there develops a three-way dynamic relationship between the child with the disability, other family members including siblings, grandparents, and any other member who has regular contact, and the outside world. This includes the local community, services, and any other place where the child with a learning disability will have contact.

Facing the future

There is evidence that increasing numbers of adults with learning disabilities are still living at home with carers who are aged over 70 (Foundation for People with Learning Disabilities 2002b). Such older carers have a range of specific needs, and these are discussed in a subsequent section. Currently families with children who have learning disabilities are encouraged to keep their child in the home environment; however, this emphasis changes as the child goes through the transition phase and becomes an adult. It is here that the adult child is encouraged to gain independence and to move away from the family home.

All the families we spoke to were concerned about future care needs and services. One family whose adult son was in his sixties felt that if he left home then they would have no focus in life, and yet they recognised that they were becoming frail themselves. They also recognised that for as much support as they gave their son, he gave them support in return in such areas as shopping, keeping the house tidy, and carrying things. This factor is discussed by Williams & Robinson (2001b) who suggests that mutual care-giving is very common in families with people who require long-term care.

The younger families expressed concerns about what would happen when their children had to leave school and enter the adult world, about whether they would leave home and where they would go. Some siblings expressed concerns about their future role in supporting their brother or sister. These factors assume greater importance as the person with learning disabilities gets older.

To conclude, the Foundation for People with Learning Disabilities (2002a) in its report *Count Us In* highlights the importance of addressing the mental health needs of young people with learning disabilities. Services need to address deficits in provision, agencies must work together to develop mental health promotion in all areas of life including schools, the workplace and at home. As the report aptly notes, '… the committee has shone a torch into a neglected area' (Foundation for People with Learning Disabilities 2002a, p 8).

Support for the older carer

The bulk of this chapter so far has focused on the needs of families of children and young people with learning disabilities and mental health problems. However, as we have noted, families in which there is a member with learning disabilities take many diverse forms, with a multitude of relationships (Grant & Ramcharan 2001), and indeed *Valuing People* (Department of Health 2001b) acknowledged the wealth of care that is provided by people who are older. These people are in their seventies, eighties and even nineties and are still caring for their dependent adult children. Often these people only come to the attention of services when there is a crisis or they acknowledge that they can no longer cope. Sometimes their struggles are never publicly revealed until one or both of the parents die.

The needs of this group of people must be identified in order to offer them the support that they require to maintain their lifestyle. Partnership boards have been tasked to meet targets in relation to older carers including:

- identifying how many older carers are aged over 70
- making sure that all clients who are cared for by an older carer have an agreed plan regarding the future
- developing systems to monitor how well services are supporting older carers.

Evidence from projects such as the GOLD (Growing Older with Learning Disabilities) programme (Foundation for People with Learning Disabilities 2002c) suggests that older carers would like to know what will happen to their child in times of emergencies, and to have confidence in the agencies who will be meeting their child's needs. Older carers, like any concerned parent, want to be informed and involved in their child's life; they wish to have flexible breaks and be able to build upon positive relationships with services that are likely to be caring for their child, either temporarily or permanently in the future.

One of the common themes expressed by the families we talked to was the fear of growing older and being unable to cope, with the realisation that somebody else would take over their role, and the fear that they would then become rejected by their child. In order to meet some of these issues, a UK government initiative – supported by a range of organisations including the British Institute of Learning Disabilities, The Home Farm Trust, Housing Options, Carers UK, and the Foundation for People with Learning Disabilities, and called 'Older Family Carers Initiative' (Foundation for People with Learning Disabilities 2002c) – was established as a 3-year project to provide support to partnership boards in identifying and meeting the needs of older carers. The initiative offered a range of inputs including consultancy to support local areas in developing services for older family carers, the dissemination of examples of good practice, the production of a newsletter, the organisation of conferences and seminars, and an evaluation of the validity of the 'Valuing People' targets for working with older carers of people with learning disabilities. Caring can be a lifelong commitment and professional carers must recognise the value of that commitment in all decisions and interventions, including contact with carers, policy development, care packages, and clients' wishes and needs.

CONCLUSION

This final chapter has attempted to draw the attention of the reader to the circumstances in which carers may find themselves when caring for someone who has both learning disabilities and a mental health problem. This chapter acknowledges that although there is an abundance of literature that informs us of the effects of learning disabilities on the family and of the effects of mental health problems on the family, less is known about the effects of their conjoint impact. We can make the assumption that if one condition causes family stress, then both conditions might produce double the amount of stress on the family, obliging the family to develop sufficient coping strategies, knowledge, and skills not only to help and support their child but also to deal with the effect of their own stress. The valuable contributions made by the families we talked to has helped us to conclude that this chapter only touches the tip of the iceberg when it comes to exploring the effects of mental health problems in learning disabilities on families. We would urge the reader to explore in more depth how families can be influential in the development of services and policy through activities such as partnership boards, representation within voluntary organisations, and above all, through listening to their children.

Finally it must be recognised that each family is unique, with its own needs, and it is the responsibility of professional carers to work with family carers to ensure that both they and their relative with learning disabilities and mental health needs receive the appropriate support and treatment to meet these unique needs.

REFERENCES

Barr O 1996 Developing services for people with learning disabilities which actively involve family members: a review of recent literature. Health and Social Care in the Community 4: 102–112

Beckman J P 1983 The influence of selected child characteristics on stress in families of handicapped infants. American Journal of Mental Deficiency 88(2): 150–156

Breslau N, Davis G C 1986 Chronic stress and major depression. Archives of General Psychiatry 43: 309–314

Bristol M M, Gallagher J J, Schopler E 1988 Mothers and fathers of young developmentally disabled and non-disabled boys: adaptation and spousal support. Developmental Psychology 24(3): 441–451

Bulger M W, Wanderman A, Goldman C R 1993 Burdens and gratifications of caregiving. Appraisal of parental care of adults with schizophrenia. American Journal of Orthopsychiatry 63(2): 255–265

Cameron S J, Dobson L A, Day D M 1991 Stress in parents of developmentally delayed and non-delayed preschool children. Canada's Mental Health, March 13–17

Clark P C, King K B 2003 Comparison of family caregivers: stroke vs persons with Alzheimer's disease. Journal of Gerontological Nursing 29(2): 45–53

Dale N 1996 Working with families of children with special needs. Partnership and practice. Routledge, London

Department of Health 2001a Family matters: counting families in. Department of Health, London

Department of Health 2001b Valuing people: a new strategy for learning disability for the 21st century. Department of Health, London

Emerson E 2003 The prevalence of psychiatric disorders in children and adolescents with and without intellectual disabilities. Journal of Intellectual Disability Research 47(1): 51–58

Emerson E, Hatton C, Felce D et al 2001 Learning disabilities: the fundamental facts. Mental Health Foundation, London

Foundation for People with Learning Disabilities 2002a Count us in: the report of the committee of inquiry into meeting the mental health needs of young people with learning disabilities. The Mental Health Foundation, London

Foundation for People with Learning Disabilities 2002b Older family carers initiative. The Mental Health Foundation, London

Foundation for People with Learning Disabilities 2002c Today and tomorrow: the report of the growing older with learning disabilities programme. The Mental Health Foundation, London

Friedrich W N, Friedrich W L 1981 Psychological assets of parents of handicapped and non-handicapped children. American Journal of Mental Deficiency 85: 551–553

Giddens A 2001 Sociology, 4th edn. Polity Press/Blackwell, Oxford

Grant G, Ramcharan P 2001 Views and experiences of people with intellectual disabilities and their families (2). The family perspective. Journal of Applied Research in Intellectual Disabilities 14: 364–380

Grant G, Whittell B 2000 Differentiated coping strategies in families with children or adults with intellectual disabilities: the relevance of gender, family composition and the life span. Journal of Applied Research in Intellectual Disabilities 13: 256–275

Heiman T 2002 Parents of children with disabilities: resilience, coping and future expectations. Journal of Developmental and Physical Disabilities 14(2): 159–171

Keitner G I, Miller I W 1990 Family functioning and major depression: an overview. American Journal of Psychiatry 147(9): 1128–1137

Marriott A, Donaldson C, Tarrier N et al 2000 Effectiveness of cognitive–behavioural family intervention in reducing the burden of care in carers of patients with Alzheimer's disease. British Journal of Psychiatry 176: 557–562

Masi G 1998 Psychiatric illness in mentally retarded adolescents: clinical features. Adolescence 33: 425–434

McIntyre L L, Blacher J, Baker B L 2002 Behavioural/mental health problems in young adults with intellectual disability: the impact on families. Journal of Intellectual Disability Research 46(3): 239–249

Norah Fry Research Centre 2002 Bridging the divide at transition. What happens for young people with learning difficulties and their families? http://www.bris.ac.uk/Depts/NorahFry/online.htm

Pejlert A 2001 Being a parent of an adult son or daughter with severe mental illness receiving professional care: parents' narratives. Health and Social Care in the Community 9(4): 194–204

Princess Royal Trust for Carers 1998 Eight hours a day and taken for granted? Cited in Department of Health 2001 Family matters: counting families in. Department of Health, London, p 9

Ryde-Brandt B 1988 Mothers of primary school children with Down's syndrome. Acta Psychiatrica Scandinavica 78: 102–108

Ryde-Brandt B 1990 Anxiety and depression in mothers of children with psychotic disorders and mental retardation. British Journal of Psychiatry 156: 118–121

Tamplin A, Goodyer I M, Herbert J 1998 Family functioning and parent general health in families of adolescents with major depressive disorder. Journal of Affective Disorders 48: 1–13

Van den Borne H W, van Hooren R H, van Gestel M et al 1999 Psychological problems, coping strategies and the need for information of parents of children with Prader–Willi syndrome and Angelman syndrome. Patient Education and Counselling 39: 205–216

Whelton C, Pawlick J 1997 Involving families in psychological rehabilitation. Psychiatric Rehabilitation Journal 20(3): 57–60

Williams R, Richardson G 1995 Together we stand: the commissioning role and management of child and adolescent mental health services. HMSO, London

Williams V, Robinson C 2001a More than one wavelength: identifying, understanding and resolving conflicts of interest between people with intellectual disability and their family carers. Journal of Applied Research in Intellectual Disabilities 14: 30–46

Williams V, Robinson C 2001b He will finish up caring for me: people with learning disabilities and mutual care. British Journal of Learning Disabilities 29: 56–62

Wilton K, Renaut J 1986 Stress levels in families with intellectually handicapped preschool children and families with non-handicapped preschool children. Journal of Mental Deficiency Research 30: 163–169

Wong D F K 2000 Stress factors and mental health of carers with relatives suffering from schizophrenia in Hong Kong: implications for culturally sensitive practice. British Journal of Social Work 30: 365–382

Wyngaarden-Krauss M 1994 Child-related and parenting stress: similarities and differences between mothers and fathers of children with disabilities. American Journal of Mental Retardation 97(4): 393–404

Yun-Hee J, Madjar I 1998 Caring for a family member with chronic mental illness. Qualitative Health Research 8(5): 694–707

Zigmond A S, Snaith R P 1983 The Hospital Anxiety and Depression Scale. Acta Psychiatrica Scandinavica 67: 361–370

Postscript

This book has attempted to bring together some of the current ideas, research, and knowledge relating to people with learning disabilities who also have a mental health problem. The book was written in the hope that carers might gain some new insights which might influence the ways in which care is delivered to this client group. We have tried to explore a wide range of issues that become relevant from the first suspicion that a person may have a mental health problem, such as how to explain and identify that problem, how to address any identified needs, and how to identify the appropriate services within the policy context which drives those services. We have sought to acknowledge the major contribution made by families across the age span, and to endorse throughout the ideology of inclusive lifestyles for people with learning disabilities who have a mental health problem.

In developing this book we have discovered many services and people that are working hard to meet the mental health needs of people with a learning disability. Throughout the UK there are countless examples of good practice ranging from individuals caring for a relative through to organisations dedicated to providing specialist care. We have discovered many examples of existing assessment tools, therapeutic interventions, and care strategies being adapted for use with this client group, as well as the development of new interventions and tools. There is also evidence that the concept of mental health problems in people with learning disabilities is being recognised and taken seriously by policy makers.

The authors of any book will recognise that there are limitations to their work, and we are no exception. As the book was developed we became conscious of the vastness of the field, and therefore recognise that this book can make only a small contribution to the care of people with learning disabilities and mental health needs. Each chapter could have been expanded, or indeed have become a book in its own right, for as we developed each chapter we discovered new ideas, services, research, and practices that could and should be addressed. The book has raised many questions, many of which cannot yet be answered fully. However, we hope that such questions, alongside the material included in this book, will have stimulated the reader to think about some possible answers. From the experiences gained in writing this book, we hope to be able to develop some of the ideas further in a subsequent publication, and thus contribute in some small way to enhancing the lives of people with learning disabilities and mental health problems.

APPENDIX 1

Communication aids

Dodd K, Gathard J 2001 Feeling poorly. Pavilion, Brighton

Fox P, Emerson E 2002 Positive goals. Interventions for people with learning disabilities whose behaviour challenges services. A resource pack. Pavilion, Brighton

Grove N 2000 See what I mean. Guidelines to aid understanding of communication by people with severe and profound learning disabilities. BILD/Mencap, Kidderminster

Hollins S, Avis A, Cheverton S 1998 Going into hospital. (Books beyond words series.) Gaskell, London

Holland A, Payne A, Vickey L 1998 Exploring your emotions (photographs and manual). BILD Publications, Plymouth

People First 2002 Access 2 pictures: a voice for people with learning disabilities. www.peoplefirst.org.uk

APPENDIX 2

Assessment and planning resources

Assessment of Dual Diagnosis (ADD): Dr J Matson, 3333 Woodland Ridge Boulevard, Baton Rouge, LA 70816, USA

Autoneed (computerised version of the Cardinal Needs Schedule) www.gac.man.ac.uk/autoneed

Brief Symptom Inventory: administration, scoring and procedures: Manual, 3rd edn. National Computer Systems, Minneapolis

Camberwell Assessment of Needs for Adults with Developmental and Intellectual Disabilities (CANDID): Section of Community Psychiatry, Institute of Psychiatry, De Crespigny Park, London SE5 8AF, UK

Dementia Questionnaire for Persons with Mental Retardation (DMR): NWO Ontginningssubsidie, Hooge Burch, PO Box 2027, 2470 AA Zwammerdam, The Netherlands

DASH-II: Dr J Matson, 3333 Woodland Ridge Boulevard, Baton Rouge, LA 70816, USA

Deb S, Matthews T, Holt G et al 2001 Practice guidelines for the assessment and diagnosis of mental health problems in adults with intellectual disability. Pavilion, Brighton (*provides references for many assessment tools/rating scales*)

Falvey M, Forster M, Pearpoint J et al 1997 All my life's a circle. Using the tools: Circles, MAPs and PATHs, 2nd edn. Inclusion Press, Toronto

Gedye Dementia Scale for Down syndrome: Gedye Research and Consulting, PO Box 39081, Vancouver, Canada

Hamilton Anxiety Scale: Online: available at www.anxietyhelp.org

Holt G, Bouras N (eds) 1997 Making links. A videotape of people with mental health needs and learning disabilities. Pavilion, Brighton

Health of the Nation Outcome Scales for Learning Disability (HoNOS-LD): BILD, Campion House, Green Street, Kidderminster DY10 1JL, UK

Hospital Anxiety and Depression (HAD) scale: A self-assessment version is available online via NHS Direct www.nhsdirect.nhs.uk

Learning Disability Version of the Cardinal Needs Schedule (LDCNS): Dr R Raghavan, School of Health Studies, Bradford University, Bradford, UK. E-mail r.raghavan@bradford.ac.uk

Mini-Mental State Examination (MMSE): www.minimental.com

PAS-ADD Instruments: Pavilion Publishing, The Ironworks, Cheapside, Brighton, BN1 4GD, UK

Reiss Screen: IDS Publishing, PO Box 389, Worthington, Ohio 43085, USA

Royal College of Psychiatrists 2001 DC-LD (Diagnostic criteria for psychiatric disorders for use with adults with learning disabilities/mental retardation). Occasional Paper OP48. Gaskell, London

Symptom Checklist 90-Revised: Administration, scoring and procedures, Manual II: Clinical Psychometric Research, Towson, MD

Xenitides K, Bouras N 2002 Measurement of needs in people with learning disabilities and mental health problems. In: Thornicroft G (ed) Measuring mental health needs, 2nd edn. Royal College of Psychiatrists, London, UK

- A range of assessment tools is available in: Schutte N, Malouff J 1995 Sourcebook of adult assessment strategies. Plenum Press, New York
- Training in the use of some tools in the UK is available from The Estia Centre, Guys Hospital, London, UK. The centre offers training to organisations that provide care and support to people with learning disabilities who have additional mental health needs or challenging behaviours. www.estiacentre.org

APPENDIX 3

Organisations

This is a selection of UK-based organisations that can provide information, services, support, advocacy, research, or training in relation to people with learning disabilities and mental health problems, their families and carers.

- BILD (British Institute of Learning Disabilities), Campion House, Green Street, Kidderminster DY10 1JL: www.bild.org.uk
- Carers UK, 20–25 Glasshouse Yard, London EC1A 4JT: www.carersonline.org.uk
- Connects: www.connects.org.uk
- Connexions: www.connexions.gov.uk
- Estia Centre: www.estiacentre.org
- Foundation for People with Learning Disabilities/The Mental Health Foundation, 83 Victoria Street, London SW1H 0HW: www.learningdisabilities.org.uk/www.mentalhealth.org.uk
- Health Evidence Bulletins Wales – Learning Disabilities: http://hebw.uwcm.ac.uk
- The Home Farm Trust: www.hft.org.uk
- Housing Options, 78a High Street, Witney, Oxon OX28 6HL: www.housingoptions.org.uk
- The Judith Trust, 5 Carriage House, 90 Randolph Avenue, London W9 1BD
- Mencap: www.mencap.org.uk
- Mind (National Association for Mental Health): www.mind.org.uk
- National Autistic Society, 393 City Road, London EC1V 1NG: www.nas.org.uk
- National Development Team: Albion Wharf, Albion Street, Manchester M1 5LN: www.ndt.org.uk
- Norah Fry Research Centre: www.bris.ac.uk/Depts/NorahFry/
- People First: www.peoplefirst.org.uk
- Recovery Movement: www.mentalhealthrecovery.org.uk
- Sainsbury Centre for Mental Health: www.scmh.org.uk

Index